Lead Poisoning
in Childhood

LEAD POISONING IN CHILDHOOD

Edited by

Siegfried M. Pueschel, M.D., Ph.D., M.P.H.

James G. Linakis, Ph.D., M.D.

Angela C. Anderson, M.D.

Rhode Island Hospital
Providence

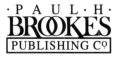

·P A U L·H·
BROOKES
PUBLISHING C?

Baltimore • London • Toronto • Sydney

Paul H. Brookes Publishing Co.
Post Office Box 10624
Baltimore, Maryland 21285-0624

Copyright © 1996 by Paul H. Brookes Publishing Co., Inc.

Typeset by Signature Typesetting & Design, Baltimore, Maryland.
Manufactured in the United States of America by
Thomson-Shore, Inc., Dexter, Michigan.

In the case studies herein, the names of the subjects have been changed to
protect their identities.

Library of Congress Cataloging-in-Publication Data
Lead poisoning in childhood / [edited by] Siegfried M. Pueschel, James G.
 Linakis, Angela C. Anderson.
      p.   cm.
   Includes bibliographical reference and index.
   ISBN 1-55766-232-0
   1. Lead poisoning in children.   2. Lead poisoning in children—
Prevention.   I. Pueschel, Siegfried, M.   II. Linakis, James G.
III. Anderson, Angela.
   [DNLM: 1. Lead Poisoning—in infancy & childhood.   QV 292 L4334
1995]
 RA 1231.L4L39   1995
 615.9′25688′083—dc20
 DNLM/DLC
 for Library of Congress   95-41441
                                                                    CIP

British Library Cataloguing-in-Publication data are available from the British
Library.

CONTENTS

Contributors

Angela C. Anderson, M.D.
Assistant Professor of Pediatrics
Brown University School
  of Medicine
Co-Director Lead Treatment Program
Rhode Island Hospital
593 Eddy Street
Providence, RI 02903

David Bellinger, Ph.D., M.Sc.
Associate Professor of Neurology
Harvard Medical School
Neuroepidemiology Unit
Children's Hospital
300 Longwood Avenue
Boston, MA 02115

Barbara Berney, M.P.H.
179 Hunnewell Avenue
Newton, MA 02158

J. Julian Chisolm, Jr., M.D.
Professor of Pediatrics
The Johns Hopkins University
Director, Lead Poisoning Program
The Kennedy Krieger Institute
707 North Broadway
Baltimore, MD 21205

Kim N. Dietrich, Ph.D.
Research Professor of Environmental
  Health
Department of Environmental Health
Division of Biostatistics and
  Epidemiology
University of Cincinnati College
  of Medicine
Cincinnati, OH 45267

Deborah E. Glotzer, M.D., M.P.H.
Assistant Professor of Pediatrics
Harvard Medical School
The Cambridge Hospital
1493 Cambridge Street
Cambridge, MA 02139

James G. Linakis, Ph.D., M.D.
Assistant Professor of Pediatrics
Brown University School
  of Medicine
Co-Director Lead Treatment Program
Rhode Island Hospital
593 Eddy Street
Providence, RI 02903

Stephanie Pollack, J.D., M.P.H.
Senior Attorney
Conservation Law Foundation
62 Summer Street
Boston, MA 02110

Siegfried M. Pueschel, M.D., Ph.D., M.P.H.
Professor of Pediatrics
Brown University School
  of Medicine
Director, Child Development Center
Rhode Island Hospital
593 Eddy Street
Providence, RI 02903

Thomas L. Schlenker, M.D., M.P.H.
Executive Director
Salt Lake City-County Health
  Department
2001 South State Street
Salt Lake City, UT 84190

Michael W. Shannon, M.D., M.P.H.
Associate Professor of Pediatrics
Harvard Medical School
Associate Chief
Division of Emergency Medicine
Children's Hospital
300 Longwood Avenue
Boston, MA 02115

Jeanne M. Solé, J.D.
Staff Attorney
Conservation Law Foundation
62 Summer Street
Boston, MA 02110

PREFACE

Since ancient times, the adverse consequences of lead exposure have plagued the human race. Even after the toxicity of lead was acknowledged, lead poisoning was thought for centuries to be primarily an occupational disease of adults, resulting from prolonged exposure to easily identifiable sources. Early in the 20th century, however, research revealed that lead's effects on children are its most pernicious.

The magnitude of childhood lead poisoning has been inexplicably neglected both by modern medicine and by legislators. Indeed, as this book was being written, nearly 2 million children in the United States were estimated to have dangerously elevated blood lead levels, making lead poisoning the nation's most prevalent preventable childhood health problem.

In spite of this tragic legacy, there is evidence that a new initiative is underway to eradicate childhood lead poisoning definitively. Interest in and understanding of lead poisoning was until recently the domain of a few individuals. Since the 1970s, however, considerably increased attention has been focused on lead poisoning in childhood, and our understanding of its implications has expanded dramatically. Advances have been made in several areas, including 1) identification of lead-poisoned patients, 2) understanding of the neurodevelopmental and behavioral ramifications of lead poisoning, 3) recognition of the consequences of low-level lead exposure, 4) remediation of sources of lead exposure, and 5) prevention and treatment of lead poisoning. Yet, as with most other disciplines, our increase in knowledge has raised at least as many questions as it has answered. Considerable work must be accomplished before we can fully understand such issues as the complete range of low-level lead effects, the most economically feasible means for effectively abating lead-based paint hazards, and the efficacy of chelation therapy in reversing lead effects.

Therefore, the purpose of this book is twofold: first, to give readers, in a concise fashion, a state-of-the-art presentation of what is known about lead poisoning in childhood; and second, and equally important, to offer critical insights into the challenges that remain in understanding lead poisoning and abolishing it as a major health problem.

We have attempted to restrict the subject matter in this book to those lead-related topics that are most relevant to *childhood* lead poisoning. Consequently, no attempt has been made to address the issue of occupational lead poisoning other than in reference to how it relates or contributes to childhood lead exposures. Chapter topics include historical perspectives on lead poisoning, epidemiology, etiology, screening, pathophysiology, behavioral concerns, lead poisoning during pregnancy, medical management, environmental abatement, legislative issues, prevention, and the economics of childhood lead poisoning.

We believe that this comprehensive coverage of the facts, effects, and implications of lead exposure will be useful to pediatricians, family physicians, pediatric nurses, social workers, child development specialists, and all health care professionals who care for children in their home and school environments. In addition, we hope that relevant sections of the book will garner the attention of environmental specialists, legislators, and project planners of enterprises centered on children's activities.

Our most important goal is to contribute to the well-being of the millions of children who continue to suffer from the devastating effects of lead poisoning. Perhaps through education at all levels and through increased public and professional awareness, the effects of centuries of ignorance and indifference can be overcome. We earnestly hope that future texts will be able to discuss childhood lead poisoning solely from a historical perspective.

LEAD POISONING
IN CHILDHOOD

1

LEAD POISONING
A HISTORICAL PERSPECTIVE

Siegfried M. Pueschel
James G. Linakis
Angela C. Anderson

L ead has been recognized as an environmental toxin since antiquity. In fact, lead poisoning is regarded as one of the earliest occupational diseases (Smith, 1986). It is presumed that many workers in ancient lead furnaces and kilns were adversely affected by inhalation of lead fumes and absorption of lead through the skin. There are reports indicating that lead poisoning likely occurred in most ancient peoples, including the Egyptians, the Greeks, and the Romans.

Since Egyptian times, lead and its compounds have been used as therapeutic agents. Greek, Roman, and Far Eastern physicians and healers used lead in various forms for medical treatments (Nriagu, 1992). On the European continent, numerous metallic drugs, including lead compounds, were used medicinally since the 16th century, and many of these therapeutic agents were later employed on the North American continent (Nriagu, 1992).

In past centuries, lead has been found to cause various ailments. For example, gastrointestinal symptoms, often referred to as *colica pictonium* and later as Devonshire colic, were apparently caused by lead poisoning (Morris, 1980). During the 19th century, specific neurologic symptoms were identified as the result of increased lead absorption.

It was only during the present century that physicians became concerned with lead poisoning in childhood. The first accounts of childhood lead poisoning in the United States were published during the 1920s (Lin-Fu, 1992). Subsequently, childhood lead poisoning was recognized as a major public health concern in this country.

EARLIEST USE OF LEAD

The use of lead dates far back in antiquity. Small beads of metallic lead have been found in excavations on the central Anatolian plain dating back to 7000–6500 B.C. (Krysko, 1979). Litharge (lead oxide) has been identified on glazed ceramics near old silver mines originating in 5000 B.C. (Krysko, 1979). The oldest known human-made lead object, most likely used for decoration, is a small carved figure of a woman from about 4000 B.C. There are many other decorative objects from about 3000–2000 B.C., such as small human and animal figurines (Smith, 1986). Metal plates made from lead were used that provide a written record from as early as 3000 B.C. In addition, Egyptians used galina (lead acetate) as a cosmetic for eye paint (Smith, 1986). Egyptians also used lead sinkers for fishing as early as 2500 B.C.

In ancient Mesopotamia, a lip salve was found dating back to 2600 B.C. Lip salves that contained lead were used by women as a cosmetic (Poucher, 1941).

The ancient Hebrews also used lead. In fact, there are several references to lead in the Old Testament. In Ezekiel 27:12, lead is mentioned in the process of cupellation; in Jeremiah 6:29–30, the process of lead production is detailed; and in Job 19:23–25, the use of lead tablets for writing is described (Smith, 1986).

As early as the fifth century B.C., metallic lead and its compounds were used as pharmaceutical agents in ancient China and other old cultures of the Far East (Nriagu, 1992). In subsequent centuries, metallic preparations containing large amounts of lead were employed in various forms for medical treatment purposes. Similarly, lead was used as a therapeutic agent in ancient India. There lead sulfite became an ingredient in "collyria," and lead oxides were prescribed with vegetable drugs for use as plasters (Nriagu, 1992).

Excavations in Troy dating back to 3000–2500 B.C. revealed artifacts of lead (Ericson, Shirahata, & Patterson, 1979). Greeks used lead vessels for making wine. Moreover, lead was often added to wine as a taste enhancer.

The Greeks had a wide variety of medications containing various lead compounds. Metallic lead, lead sulfite, and various lead oxides were used in therapeutic applications. For example, the Hippocratic collection had about 30 medications containing lead oxides. Galen and Celsus, as well as their disciples, used numerous lead compounds as antiseptics, as applications for ulcers, and to control bleeding (Nriagu, 1992).

ROMAN PERIOD

In the third century B.C., Greek medicine was introduced in Rome. Eventually, the Romans developed an impressive lead technology and used lead more extensively than any other civilization before it. The Roman aqueducts were lined with lead sheets, many cooking utensils were coated with a mixture of lead and silver, and lead vessels were used for wine production and as ornaments. The main use of lead in the Roman Empire was in sanitary engineering. The Romans had an elaborate system of piping and cisterns that supplied water to towns and houses throughout the Roman Empire. These pipes and cisterns were made from cast lead sheets (Nriagu, 1992).

In addition, the Romans used lead sheets for roofing, made ship anchors and ship keels out of lead, and used lead for coin making. Another use included lead compounds as pigments for coloring.

It is assumed that many of the ancient artisans who worked in lead mines probably had lead poisoning, as mentioned above. It has been estimated that the number of workers who were exposed to lead was over 140,000 per year during the time of the Roman Empire. The process of lead smelting and refining was often associated with a high level of exposure to toxic lead fumes (Nriagu, 1983).

According to Nriagu (1983), the population living near the smelting facilities and lead mines also had a high exposure to lead. It must be presumed that the noxious lead dust and fumes generated by the smelters rained on inhabitants and contaminated their cisterns. Moreover, workers in such industries as plumbing, roofing, and pottery glazing must have been exposed to lead and thus were at high risk for lead poisoning (Nriagu, 1983). Many of these workers probably contaminated their home environment with lead dust brought home on their clothing and thus exposed other family members to lead. Nriagu (1983) points out that, in spite of the high exposure to lead in smelters, mines, and other workplaces, there is no evidence in the Roman literature that occupational lead poisoning was recognized at that time.

Aside from industrial sources of lead poisoning, the principal source of ingested lead for affluent Romans was sapa, a boiled-down grape syrup. The boiling down process was typically performed in a lead pot or lead-lined copper kettle. According to Patterson, Shirahata, and Ericson (1987), sapa was an ingredient added to wine just before it was sealed in amphorae. The additive was intended to prevent contamination by bacteria and yeast and to prevent the wine from becoming sour. In effect, the lead in sapa acted as a fungicide and bactericide that impeded fermentation and oxidation. In addition, sapa was thought to enhance the color, sweetness, and bouquet of the wine.

The Romans apparently had a taste for wine. The average daily consumption of Roman wine drinkers was estimated to be about 1–5 L (Hofmann, 1883). Thus, the intake of lead by aristocrats in the Roman Empire was remarkable. Indeed, the Roman aristocracy ingested more than enough lead in their wine each day—approximately 250 µg—to put them at high risk for lead poisoning. It is not surprising, then, that a Roman physician, Paul of Aegina, reported an "epidemic of lead poisoning" during the seventh century A.D. He described intestinal symptoms resembling colic in numerous individuals, many of whom became "epileptics and had temporal paralysis of the lower extremities" (Steinbock, 1979, p. 277).

MEDIEVAL PERIOD

During medieval times, the old lead mines in England, which originally were exploited by the Romans, were reopened as a result of the demand for lead for both roofing and piping. In 1285, for example, lead pipes were laid in Cheapside in the city of London to supply the city with water piped in from outside the city (Smith, 1986). Lead was also used in large church glass windows to hold pieces of colored glass together. Moreover, lead was a very fashionable material for a wide variety of statues and monuments (Smith, 1986).

Medieval people apparently were cognizant of the sources and manifestations of lead poisoning. According to Green (1985), during the 15th century, both the French and Spanish governments issued decrees prohibiting the addition of lead compounds to wine. By the end of the 15th century, in some parts of Germany, the addition of lead to wine was also prohibited.

Nevertheless, during the Middle Ages, many physicians and pharmacists recommended lead in various forms of pharmaceutical treatment. Advocated by Paracelsus in the 16th century, lead acetate was frequently used for a wide variety of diseases. The 1698 *Dispensatorium Brandenburgicum* recommended both lead sulfate and lead acetate for treatment purposes. Lead acetate was often used in monasteries as an antiaphrodisiac, which apparently resulted in lead poisoning of epidemic proportions (Nriagu, 1992). Lead was also employed for internal bleeding. At the end of the 17th century, Pomet recommended lead acetate for intestinal and upper respiratory ailments (Nriagu,

1992). These are but a few examples of the widespread use of lead for a variety of conditions.

LEAD POISONING DURING THE LAST FEW CENTURIES

Although intestinal symptoms often described as "colic" have been reported in the literature since Roman times, only during the past few centuries has it become evident that colic was caused by lead-containing alcoholic beverages. Citois was probably the first physician to observe that colic was secondary to lead poisoning (Morris, 1980). Citois described an epidemic of colic that took place in Poitou in 1572, often referred to as *Colica Pictonium*. The origin of lead-induced colic was ultimately traced to the practice of adding lead oxide to sour wines. Similar gastrointestinal ailments had also been observed in other countries. For example, colic was described as "entrapado" in Spain, the "Huttenkatze" in Germany, the "bellain" of Derbyshire, the "colic of Devonshire" in England, and the "dry bellyache" in the United States (Waldron, 1973).

At the end of the 17th century, the German physician Gockel was struck by epidemics of colic in southern Germany. At that time, many towns in Swabia used lead acetate to sweeten sour wines. Gockel, alerted by colic outbreaks in two monasteries in southern Germany, identified the connection between sweetening of acid wine with litharge and the intestinal symptoms, which prior to that time often went undiagnosed (Eisinger, 1982).

In the Americas, rum was frequently imported that had been distilled in lead pipes and therefore contained high concentrations of lead. Individuals who drank rum often suffered from "dry gripes." In 1745, Benjamin Franklin became interested in this subject and discussed the "West India dry gripes" in a letter to Dr. Evans and, later, with his friend Vaughan. In these letters, Franklin expressed his insight into the pathogenesis of lead poisoning due to the increased lead content in rum (Felton, 1967).

Sir George Baker described the Devonshire colic in 1767. He had noted that people with intestinal symptoms of colic usually drank cider made in Devonshire presses, which were lined with lead. Once the lead linings were removed from the cider presses, colic was less often observed (Waldron, 1970).

In 1839, Tranquerel des Planches published his book on diseases of lead in which he described more than 1,000 patients with lead poisoning and secondary gastrointestinal and neurologic symptoms (Beritic, 1989). Des Planches felt that abdominal pain is the most important symptom and, together with constipation, characterized lead-induced colic. He noted abdominal guarding, rigidity, and tenderness in the majority of patients with lead-induced colic.

Although there were probably many causes of lead poisoning, improperly prepared glazing compounds, alcoholic beverages that contained lead, and pewter drinking utensils may have been the most common sources of lead in humans.

During the latter half of the 19th century, attempts were made to overcome the problem of lead poisoning in England. At that time, lead poisoning was prevalent among glazemakers, dippers, and their assistants working with earthenware and china. Many of these individuals experienced colic, convulsions, paralysis of limbs, and blindness. Moreover, female lead workers often had miscarriages. The government soon became concerned, and in 1883 the Factory Prevention of Lead Poisoning Act was passed. In August 1900, the secretary of state in London issued a draft providing special rules to prevent lead poisoning. In 1913, the Regulation for the Manufacture and Decoration of Pottery Act was introduced. These regulations restricted the employment of women, young persons, and children in various manufacturing processes that involved lead. The act also mandated the use of protective clothing, proper storage facilities for outdoor garments, and the suppression of dust in an attempt to limit the inhalation of lead fumes (Morris, 1980).

Other countries also enacted legislation to prevent lead poisoning during the early 20th century. For example, Germany has controlled the lead content in paint since 1900. In France, regulations prohibiting the use of lead-containing paint on toys and on walls of living quarters have been enforced since 1915 (Pueschel & Fadden, 1975). As early as 1922, the nations participating in the International Labor Office in Geneva proposed to disallow the application of white lead paint in the interior of buildings. Also in 1922, physicians in Australia initiated a campaign that led to the introduction of laws restricting the use of lead paint in that country (Failey, 1934; Pueschel & Fadden, 1975). Countries such as Tunisia, Greece, Sweden, Great Britain, Belgium, Spain, and Poland also introduced legislation that prohibited lead-based paint in the interior of buildings during the first half of this century (Rabin, 1989).

CHILDHOOD LEAD POISONING

Although there have been sporadic reports of lead poisoning in children during past centuries, primarily as a consequence of secondary occupational lead exposure, childhood lead poisoning was first recognized as a separate entity at the turn of the 20th century. The earliest reports of childhood lead poisoning were provided by Australian physicians. Turner (1897) described lead poisoning in children as "toxicity of habitation" because symptoms of lead poisoning often recurred after children had been released from the hospital to their homes. However, the source of lead poisoning remained a mystery until the early 1900s. In 1904, Gibson suggested that lead paint, in particular paint at railings and walls, was the source of lead poisoning among affected Queensland, Australia, children. In addition, Gibson made other important observations such as the seasonal occurrence of lead poisoning, nail biting, sucking of fingers, and eating with unwashed hands in children who were found to have lead poisoning.

In the United States, the first reports on childhood lead poisoning were published during the second decade of the 20th century. In 1914, Thomas and Blackfan reported a child with central nervous system insult due to lead poisoning. Three years later Blackfan (1917) pointed out that patients with convulsive disorders of unknown origin should be suspected of having lead poisoning.

During the 1920s, lead poisoning was more often recognized in children than before. Ruddock (1924) suggested that there are many children who present with a mild form of lead poisoning involving intestinal symptoms such as spasms or colic. He concluded that "a child lives in a lead world." Similarly, McKhann (1933) was convinced that lead poisoning is a relatively frequent occurrence in young children.

During the 1930s, a number of case reports were published pointing to lead paint on the interior of houses as the source of lead poisoning (Blackman, 1937; Cushing, 1934; Donnally, Schutz, & Nimetz, 1935). These reports often described symptoms of lead poisoning such as abdominal pain, constipation, irritability, and vomiting as well as neurologic signs (Rabin, 1989). Because the source of lead poisoning was well identified, many physicians who were involved in the care of children with lead poisoning attempted to ban the use of lead paint in the interior of homes.

In the 1930s, the Baltimore Health Department played a leading role in developing the first extensive public health program to prevent childhood lead paint poisoning (Fee, 1990). In 1935, a free blood lead laboratory service for physicians and hospitals was initiated that could be utilized by physicians for screening purposes (Baltimore Health Department, 1971).

Although it was well known by that time that lead paint was the main culprit causing lead poisoning in children, there were no significant efforts in the United States to reduce or eliminate the lead in paint in the first half of the 20th century. The lead industry was aware of the dangers that lead paint posed to young children (McKhann & Vogt, 1933), yet it ignored or suppressed such information. Furthermore, investigators and physicians dealing with childhood lead poisoning, some of whom were closely associated with and/or funded by the lead industry, did not forcefully communicate to the industry the importance of eliminating lead from paint. Even during the 1940s, when more reports on lead poisoning were published indicating lead paint as the main cause of lead poisoning in children, the lead industry often denied the significance of the problem. Industry representatives either discredited such reports or downplayed the lead poisoning problem. In addition, the lead industry intimidated physicians working in the field of childhood lead poisoning by threatening legal action (Rabin, 1989).

The paint industry claimed that the use of lead in paint intended for interior application was discontinued by 1940. However, lead paint continued to be produced. Rabin (1989) reported that as late as 1971 there was evidence of significant amounts of lead paint being sold for residential interior use. Thus, in spite of the lead industry's claims, the practice of covering interior surfaces with lead-based paint continued in the decades after 1940.

During the 1960s, lead poisoning was increasingly recognized as an important pediatric public health problem. Many cities started to screen children for lead poisoning during the 1960s, 1970s, and 1980s. Chicago was one of the first cities where mass screening was pursued (Blanksma, Sachs, & Murray, 1969). Shortly thereafter other cities, such as Baltimore, New York, Philadelphia, and Boston, initiated lead poisoning screening programs. By the 1970s, the U.S. Surgeon General issued a statement on the problem of childhood lead poisoning and recommended early identification of children with undue lead absorption (Surgeon General, 1971).

Whereas many other countries had initiated legislative action with regard to lead poisoning in the beginning of the 20th century, it was not until the late 1960s that the United States introduced legislation to provide federal assistance to local governments for projects involving the detection and treatment of lead poisoning in children (HR 9192, 1969). Federal funds were allocated for rehabilitation of older houses and to encourage cities and communities to develop intensive local programs to eliminate the health hazards of lead-based paint poisoning (S 3216, 1969). After a drawn-out legislative process including hearings and discussions in various committees, a compromise bill, the Lead-Based Paint Poisoning Prevention Act, was passed by both House and Senate in the late 1970s and signed into law by the president in January 1971 (PL 91-695, 1971). The act authorized grants up to 75% of the total cost of local programs for the detection and treatment of lead-based paint poisoning. In conjunction with this program, grants were also authorized to assist local governments in identifying housing units in which lead-based paint surfaces constituted a health hazard.

Unfortunately, programs authorized by this act never gained momentum. The main reasons were the apparent indifference of the Nixon administration to childhood lead poisoning and a significant reduction of appropriations. The Lead-Based Paint Poisoning Prevention Act expired on June 19, 1972, despite attempts in Congress to extend it (Pueschel & Fadden, 1975).

During the 93rd Congress, new legislation was introduced to extend and amend the previous law. Both Senate and House reports recommended adoption of legislation that would expand the Lead-Based Paint Poisoning Prevention Act. A revised version of the act was passed in both houses and signed into law in November 1973 (PL 93-151, 1973). An important change in the law was the increase of federal support from the original 75%–90% for programs relating to the detection and treatment of childhood lead poisoning. This legislation took a stronger position on environmental conditions than the previous law. The Secretary of Housing and Urban Development was to establish procedures to eliminate the hazards of lead-based paint in older housing units. The law also prohibited application of lead-based paint to federally funded residential structures and outlawed the use of lead-based paint on toys, furniture, and cooking utensils. In addition, research and demonstration programs were to focus on the deleading of housing units. Although the Senate had authorized $75 million and the House $52 million for fiscal years 1974 and 1975, only 8% of this sum was actually appropriated for fiscal year 1974.

State legislatures also became aware of the increased risk to children of lead-based paint in older inner-city dwellings, and many states initiated laws to prevent this human-made disease. For example, based on a case study carried out in an impoverished section of Boston in 1968 (Pueschel, Kopito, & Shwachman, 1972) as well as other evidence of the high risk of lead-based paint to children, four bills on lead poisoning prevention were brought before the Massachusetts legislature by the spring of 1971. After hearings, committee reviews, and routine legislative maneuvers, the Senate and the House approved the bill originally drafted by the Massachusetts Law Reform Institute. In

November 1971, the Lead Poisoning Prevention and Control Act was passed by both houses and subsequently signed into law by the governor (Mass. Gen. Laws Ann. ch. 111, §§ 189A et seq., 1971).

The Massachusetts law required the establishment of a statewide program for prevention, screening, diagnosis, and treatment of lead poisoning. Public health personnel were required to report cases within 3 days of discovery to the director of the program, who then had to disseminate this information to the local boards of health and enforcement agencies. An important aspect of this program dealt with the detection of sources of lead poisoning, in particular those dwellings where children are exposed to lead-containing paint. It was emphasized that all children in such dwellings who are under the age of 6 years should be screened for lead poisoning. The law acknowledged that the major threat to children comes from interior surfaces of houses covered with lead-based paint and that the removal of such paint from the environment is an important objective. The owners of residential properties where children under 6 years of age reside were obliged to remove or adequately cover any paint or plaster containing dangerous levels of lead. Failure of the landlord to remove lead-based paint was to be treated as a violation of the sanitary code. Legally, this allowed the code enforcement agency to initiate criminal prosecution (Pueschel & Fadden, 1975). Thus, Massachusetts instituted one of the most comprehensive laws concerning lead poisoning in childhood in the United States, and many other states followed suit.

Although progress has been made on both the federal and state levels regarding lead poisoning legislation, many children are still suffering the consequences of inadequate funding and governmental inertia. Concerned citizens, including physicians, question why the progress achieved has taken so long. As early as 1786, Benjamin Franklin, in a letter to his friend Vaughan, discussed the "mischievous effects of lead," wisely predicting, "You will observe with concern, how long a useful truth may be known and exist, before it is generally received and practiced on" (Felton, 1967, p. 548).

In addition to important legislative initiatives during the past decades, numerous studies have been carried out that focused on the etiology and epidemiology of lead poisoning as well as on the neurodevelopment of children with "low" levels of lead. We have also learned of the effects of lead poisoning on behavior, academic achievement, and cognitive function in children and of the toxic effects of lead on the fetus (Lin-Fu, 1992). In addition, new treatment modalities have been investigated in the 1990s.

Significant changes have taken place since the 1960s with respect to "acceptable" blood lead levels. In the early 1960s, it had been generally assumed that the upper "normal" blood lead level in adults was about 80 µg/dL and in children 60 µg/dL, respectively. In the mid-1960s, it was suggested that the upper limit for children's blood lead levels should be lowered to 40 µg/dL, which was finally accomplished in 1970. In 1975, the Centers for Disease Control reduced the upper limit of blood lead levels to 30 µg/dL, 10 years later to 25 µg/dL, and in 1991 to 10 µg/dL (Lin-Fu, 1992).

In spite of the achievements and the progress made during the past decades in the identification and treatment of childhood lead poisoning, we have not yet eradicated this human-made disease. As detailed in this chapter, lead has caused significant health concerns since ancient times. By learning from history and applying our present knowledge, we should be able to prevent the occurrence of lead poisoning, treat appropriately those children who are affected, and provide an environment that is safe and free of lead-containing materials so that children will be able to enjoy a better quality of life.

REFERENCES

Baltimore Health Department. (1971). Chronology of lead poisoning control: Baltimore 1931–71. *Baltimore Health News*, 34–40.

Beritic, T. (1989). Spinal origin of human lead neuropathy: This paper marks the 150th anniversary of Paralysie de Plomb ou Saturnine. *American Journal of Industrial Medicine, 15,* 643–656.

Blackfan, K.D. (1917). Lead poisoning in children with especial reference to lead as a cause of convulsions. *American Journal of Medical Science, 153,* 877–887.

Blackman, S.S. (1937). The lesions of lead encephalitis in children. *Bulletin of the Johns Hopkins Hospital, 61,* 1–61.

Blanksma, L.A., Sachs, H.K., & Murray, E.F. (1969). Incidence of high blood-lead levels in Chicago children. *Pediatrics, 44,* 661–667.

Cushing, H.B. (1934). Lead poisoning in children. *International Clinics, 1,* 189–191.

Donnally, H.H., Schutz, C.A., & Nimetz, A. (1935). Chronic lead poisoning in early childhood. *Virginia Medicine, 62,* 83–89.

Eisinger, J. (1982). Lead and wine: Eberhard Gockel and the colica pictonium. *Medical History, 26,* 279–302.

Ericson, J.E., Shirahata, H., & Patterson, C.C. (1979). Skeletal concentrations of lead in ancient Peruvians. *New England Journal of Medicine, 300,* 946–951.

Failey, K.D. (1934). A review of the evidence relating to lead as an etiological agent in chronic nephritis in Queensland. *Medical Journal of Australia, 1,* 600–606.

Fee, E. (1990). Public health in practice: An early confrontation with the "silent epidemic" of childhood lead paint poisoning. *Journal of the History of Medicine and Allied Sciences, 45,* 570–606.

Felton, J.S. (1967). Man, medicine and work in America: An historical series, III. Benjamin Franklin and his awareness of lead poisoning. *Journal of Occupational Medicine, 9,* 543–554.

Gibson, J.L. (1904). A plea for painted railings and painted walls of rooms as the source of lead poisoning among Queensland children. *Australian Medical Gazette, 23,* 149–153.

Green, D.W. (1985). The Saturnine curse: A history of lead poisoning. *Southern Medical Journal, 78,* 48–51.

Hofmann, K.B. (1883). Die Getränke der Griechen und Römer vom hygienischen Standpunkte. *Archiv der Geschichte der Medizin, 6,* 26–35.

HR 9192, 91st Cong., 1st Sess. (1969).

Krysko, W.W. (1979). *Lead in history and art.* Stuttgart, Germany: Rieder-Verlag.

Lead-Based Paint Poisoning Prevention Act, PL 91-695 (Jan. 13, 1971). Title 42, U.S.C. §§ 4801 et seq.: *U.S. Statutes at Large, 84,* 2078–2080.

Lead-Based Paint Poisoning Prevention Act Amendments, PL 93-151. (November 9, 1973). Title 42, U.S.C. §§ 4821–4822, *U.S. Statutes at Large, 87,* 560–568.

Lin-Fu, J.S. (1992). Modern history of lead poisoning: A century of discovery and rediscovery. In H.L. Needleman (Ed.), *Human lead exposure* (pp. 23–43). Boca Raton, FL: CRC Press.

Mass. Gen. Laws Ann., ch. 111, §§ 189A et seq. (West 1971).

McKhann, C. (1933). Lead poisoning in children: Cerebral manifestations. *Archives of Neurology, 27,* 294–304.

McKhann, C., & Vogt, E. (1933). Lead poisoning in children. *Journal of the American Medical Association, 101,* 1131–1135.

Morris, E. (1980). Lead poisoning: An historic overview. *Occupational Health, 32,* 449–459.

Nriagu, J.O. (1983). Occupational exposure to lead in ancient times. *The Science of the Total Environment, 31,* 105–116.

Nriagu, J.O. (1992). Saturnine drugs and medical exposure to lead: An historic outline. In H.L. Needleman (Ed.), *Human lead exposure* (pp. 3–21). Boca Raton, FL: CRC Press.

Patterson, C.C., Shirahata, H., & Ericson, J.E. (1987). Lead in ancient human bones and its relevance to historical developments of social problems with lead. *The Science of the Total Environment, 61,* 167–200.

Poucher, W.A. (1941). *Perfumes, cosmetics, and soaps* (6th ed.). London: Chapman & Hall.

Pueschel, S.M., & Fadden, M.E. (1975). Childhood lead poisoning and legislative action. *Journal of Legal Medicine, 3,* 16–20.

Pueschel, S.M., Kopito, L., & Shwachman, H. (1972). Children with an increased lead burden: A screening and follow-up study. *Journal of the American Medical Association, 222,* 462–466.

Rabin, R. (1989). Warnings unheeded: A history of childhood lead poisoning. *American Journal of Public Health, 79,* 1668–1674.

Ruddock, J. (1924). Lead poisoning in children. *Journal of the American Medical Association, 82,* 1682–1684.

S 3216, 91st Cong., 1st Sess. (1969).

Smith, M. (1986). Lead in history. In R. Lansdown & W. Yule (Eds.), *Lead toxicity: History and environmental impact* (pp. 7–24). Baltimore: Johns Hopkins University Press.

Steinbock, R.T. (1979). Lead ingestion in history. *New England Journal of Medicine, 301,* 277.

Stevenson, L.G. (1949). *History of lead poisoning.* Doctoral thesis, Johns Hopkins University, Baltimore, MD.

Surgeon General, U.S. Public Health Service. (1971). Medical aspects of child-hood lead poisoning. *Pediatrics, 48,* 464.

Thomas, H.M., & Blackfan, K.D. (1914). Recurrent meningitis, due to lead, in a child of five years. *American Journal of Diseases in Children, 8,* 377.

Turner, A.J. (1897). Lead poisoning among Queensland children. *Australian Medical Gazette, 16,* 475–487.

Waldron, H.A. (1970). The Devonshire colic. *Journal of History of Medicine, 25,* 383–413.

Waldron, H.A. (1973). Lead poisoning in the ancient world. *Medical History, 17,* 391–399.

2

Epidemiology of Childhood Lead Poisoning

Barbara Berney

"**L**ead is toxic wherever it is found, and it is found everywhere."
Thus the Agency for Toxic Substances and Disease Registry's 1988 report on lead poisoning in children (ATSDR, 1988) neatly summarized the previous 25 years of epidemiologic and toxicologic studies of lead.

Lead has been a known poison for thousands of years (see also Chapter 1). The ancient Greeks described the classical signs and symptoms of lead poisoning, such as colic, constipation, pallor, and palsy (Lin-Fu, 1980). Some historians suggest that Roman use of lead acetate to process wine contributed to the fall of the empire (Mack, 1973). Despite its known toxicity, lead use in the United States increased enormously from the industrial revolution through the 1970s, especially after World War II. Between 1940 and 1977, the annual consumption of lead in the United States almost doubled to 1,505,000 tons (Lin-Fu, 1982). Beginning in the 1980s, the regulation of lead in gasoline—leading to its virtual elimination as a gasoline additive—led to a decrease in total lead use in the United States and a consequent and significant decrease in population blood lead levels (Piomelli & Wolff, 1994).

Since 1950, the number of children recognized to be at risk of developing cognitive and neurobehavioral damage from lead exposure has grown dramatically. Continuing careful epidemiologic studies of the health effects of lead have demonstrated neurobehavioral and other effects at increasingly lower blood lead levels. Since 1950, the blood lead level at which studies have observed health effects has fallen from 80 µg/dL to 10 µg/dL. At the same time, lead has come to be recognized as a ubiquitous toxin presenting a hazard in soil, dust, air, and water, as well as in more traditional sources such as paint. The lowered acceptable blood lead levels combined with an increased dispersion of lead in the environment have expanded the population at risk (those with blood lead levels ≥10 µg/dL) to include 1.7 million (or almost 9% of) children in the United States under 6 years of age (Brody et al., 1994). No other health problem affects so many children in the United States. Some 0.5% of all children ages 1–5 years and 1.4% of non-Hispanic black children in this age range have blood lead levels of 25 µg/dL or greater. By contrast, a combined total of 36,000 cases of Lyme disease, measles, mumps, tuberculosis, and chicken pox was reported in children under 9 years of age (affecting less than 0.2% of children under age 9) in 1993 ("Blood lead levels," 1994).

The population at greatest risk for lead poisoning was accurately defined in 1951, when the Baltimore Health Department (1971) completed a study of 293 children with lead poisoning that occurred from 1931 to 1951. The results showed that lead poisoning occurred most often in 2-year-olds and that incidence was greatly increased during the summer months. The children "lived in old rented properties and ate paint flakes or chewed on windowsills." These demographics and case characteristics were confirmed in studies carried out in other cities such as New York and Philadelphia, as well as in larger studies performed over the subsequent 30 years. Thus, the population at greatest risk, the source of the lead, and the seasonal variation of lead poisoning incidence were all identified in the early 1950s (Eidsvold, Mustalish, & Novick, 1974). Each of these studies stressed the importance of eliminating lead paint from children's environment as the key to both effective prevention and treatment. Neither the population at greatest risk for lead poisoning nor the prescription for elimination of lead from children's environments has changed significantly since then.

What has changed over time is the understanding of lead's health effects and the blood lead levels at which these effects occur. This new knowledge has, in turn, affected the Centers for Disease Control's (CDC's) blood lead action level, the sources of lead considered significant, and the scope and number of children considered to be at risk. These changes are discussed in this chapter.

EFFECTS OBSERVED AT LOWER BLOOD LEAD LEVELS

As mentioned earlier, increasingly careful studies of lead's effects on children have led to recognition of effects at lower and lower blood lead levels and a growing population of children recognized to be at risk. The at-risk population has expanded, not just in numbers, but in the class, race, and geographic location of the people affected. As the affected population expanded and lower blood levels were considered hazardous, and as the understanding of the cumulative effects of exposure grew, the sources of exposure considered important also changed and expanded. In the 1950s and 1960s, consumption of deteriorating lead-based paint was regarded as the primary cause of lead poisoning. Public health and medical professionals believed that lead poisoning was a problem predominantly affecting poor minority children in eastern and midwestern inner cities, the so-called lead belt (Lin-Fu, 1979). But as increasing numbers of children were found to have elevated blood lead levels and the definition of *undue absorption* fell, research focused on additional sources of lead, including lead paint on intact surfaces as well as lead in gasoline, soil, dust, water, and food. The newer sources of concern existed throughout the United States and affected children of every class and color (Berney, 1993).

Until the mid- to late 1960s, lead poisoning was viewed as an acute disease leading to encephalopathy and was diagnosed in its earlier stages only by suspicious and informed physicians. Blood lead levels in diagnosed children generally exceeded 80 µg/dL and were often well above 100 µg/dL (see also Chapter 1). Although clinical case finding in the 1950s and early 1960s was based on the identification of overt symptoms of lead poisoning, investigators began looking for neurologic sequelae of lead exposure (Berney, 1993; Byers, 1959; Mellins & Jenkins, 1955; Perlstein & Attala, 1966). Their studies included children with relatively mild symptoms of poisoning. The evidence suggested that even low blood lead levels in apparently asymptomatic children might cause subtle central nervous system (CNS) effects. These findings led clinicians and public health officials to recommend that the definition of "normal" blood lead levels be lowered. In the 1950s, one group in Baltimore recommended that the definition of normal blood lead level in children be reduced from 60–80 µg/dL to 50 µg/dL. In the 1960s, this group again proposed lowering the definition of normal blood lead from 60 µg/dL to 40 µg/dL (Lin-Fu, 1970, 1972).

Several researchers working in the 1950s studied the neurologic sequelae of lead poisoning. Mellins and Jenkins (1955) investigated the mental and emotional development of a cohort of Chicago children hospitalized for lead poisoning. They found that extreme irritability, fearfulness, weakness, withdrawal, and crying for no apparent reason preceded hospitalization in many children. These symptoms suggested CNS effects. They also reported speech problems, especially related to naming of objects and conceptualization, which would "limit the symbolic processes so necessary to mature verbal behavior"; problems with visual motor coordination, especially fine motor coordination; distractibility; and short attention span. These symptoms and effects occurred during or after hospitalization or on follow-up examinations and suggested virtually all the subtle damage reported in much later studies of low-level exposure. The Chicago study and one completed by Smith (1954), which came to virtually identical conclusions, considered 50–60 µg/dL to be normal blood lead levels and 70–80 µg/dL as levels indicative of frank lead poisoning.

In 1959, Byers cited the findings noted above and suggested that lead poisoning might be a much bigger problem than the available data indicated. He observed that some lead poisoning might be due, not to pica, but rather to the normal mouthing of children in environments where paint contained very high levels of lead. He noted that intact paint as well as peeling paint could represent a hazard. He reported that some researchers had noted that lead poisoning might occur at blood levels as low as 40 µg/dL. He further reported the presence of lead in cord blood of gestationally exposed neonates and in infants less than 6 months of age. He also suggested that chronic exposure or reexposure to lead after treatment appeared to result in greater risk of mental retardation than single or short-term high-dose exposure that was properly, adequately, and quickly treated (Byers, 1959).

Screening programs begun in the 1960s led to the "discovery" of large numbers of children with lead poisoning. In New York City, only 116 children with lead poisoning were reported in 1958; 700 were reported in 1968–1969. The screening carried out in several large cities from 1967 to 1970 showed that 25%–45% of 1- to 6-year-old children from high-risk areas had blood lead levels exceeding 40 µg/dL, which was considered at the time to be the maximum acceptable level (Lin-Fu, 1979). "Most of these children had no symptoms of lead poisoning. Suddenly, undue lead absorption unassociated with overt clinical evidence of toxicity gained recognition as a phenomenon which required careful investigation because of the enormous number of young children involved" (Lin-Fu, 1979).

In 1970, the U.S. Surgeon General issued a statement that shifted the focus in lead poisoning from case finding and treatment of overt lead poisoning to its prevention through mass screening of young children and the termination of hazardous exposure for those with evidence of undue lead absorption (U.S. Department of Health, Education, and Welfare, 1970). It defined *undue exposure* as a blood lead level of 40 µg/dL at a time when 45% of the children screened in New York City had blood lead levels above this value (USDHEW, 1970). The burden on local health departments was immense. This blood lead level, considered to be asymptomatic at the time, was chosen as an action level in order to allow time to remove a child from leaded surroundings before undue exposure led to poisoning. Lin-Fu (personal communication, April 19, 1990), who helped write the Surgeon General's statement, remarked that one does not wait to remove known poisons until symptoms occur, but rather removes them as soon as evidence of ingestion occurs. The epidemiologic work of the 1960s provided new and expanded information on the effects of lead on children, the blood lead levels at which these effects might occur, and the number of children exposed. This information was used to push for new policies on controlling lead exposure and implementing intervention programs. The agitation, epidemiology, and publicity of the late 1960s led to not only the Surgeon General's statement but also congressional hearings on lead poisoning and the passage of the Lead-Based Paint Poisoning Prevention Act of 1971 (PL 91-695). Under the act, the CDC funded the screening of close to 4 million children from 1972 to 1981 (Lin-Fu, 1985).

In the early 1970s, biologic and epidemiologic findings on lead absorption and lead's effect on enzyme systems and the CNS led to greatly increased concern about low-level lead exposure in children. In 1972, King, Schaplowsky, and McCabe suggested that children might absorb lead from the intestinal tract more efficiently than adults. A year earlier, King (1971) had estimated the "maximum safe daily dose" at 300 µg of lead from all sources, assuming absorption of 10% of ingested lead. By 1974, at least one study had confirmed that children absorbed close to 50% of the lead they ingested (Alexander, 1974). These new findings represented a quintupling of the presumed absorption rate for children. Thus, the amount of lead that a child needed to consume in order to raise blood lead to the level of concern was less than previously thought. These findings led to a change in thinking about the importance of pica in cases of undue lead absorption (Lin-Fu, 1973; Sayre, Charney, & Vostal, 1974). It was suggested and confirmed that normal hand-to-mouth activity in normal ambient environments could cause undue exposure. Several studies found that aminolevulinic acid dehydratase showed a continuous dose response to blood lead levels from 5 µg/dL to 95 µg/dL (Hernberg & Nikkanen, 1970; Hernberg, Nikkanen, Mellen, & Lilius, 1970; Millar, Cummings, Battistini, Carswell, & Goldberg, 1970; Secchi, Erba, & Cambiaghi,

1974). Retrospective studies suggested that mental retardation and learning disabilities occurred in children previously considered asymptomatic (de la Burde & Choate, 1972, 1975; Perino & Ernhart, 1974; Rummo, 1974). In 1973, an article appeared in the *Journal of the American Medical Association* comparing blood lead levels in rural and urban populations and suggesting that 40 µg/dL might be too high for a definition of *undue absorption* (Cohen, Bowers, & Lepow, 1973). The authors referred to other studies of screened children and articles on hyperactivity in children with low-level lead exposure that had appeared in *Lancet* the previous year (David, Clark, & Voeller, 1972). Although these findings were challenged, they stimulated additional research on CNS effects at low exposure levels. In 1975, the CDC lowered the intervention level to 30 µg/dL.

Ten years later, in 1985, the CDC again changed the definition of *elevated blood lead level* from 30 µg/dL to 25 µg/dL, effectively doubling the number of children defined as *at risk* (CDC, 1985). This decision was based on studies showing "that lower levels of exposure may cause serious behavioral and biochemical changes" (CDC, 1985, p. 3). Studies found neurologic dysfunctions in children at increasingly lower lead levels. De la Burde and Choate (1972) observed neurologic dysfunction in children above 30 µg/dL, with a mean blood lead of 59 µg/dL. In a follow-up study on the same children (1975), the authors found evidence of persistent neurological involvement and a greatly increased rate of school failure and school problems. These and other case reference studies performed in the 1970s matched cases and controls by race and other social and economic variables (de la Burde & Choate, 1975; Kotok, Kotok, & Heriot, 1977; Rummo, 1974).

The Needleman et al. (1979) study of mostly white schoolchildren in Chelsea and Somerville, Massachusetts, was a landmark investigation of neurobehavioral effects of low-level lead exposure. All of his subjects came from English-speaking households. Needleman and co-workers collected shed deciduous teeth from 2,146 children and analyzed them for lead content. Controlling for 39 confounding variables, they found lead-affected cognitive function and adaptive classroom behavior. Needleman et al. did not collect blood samples from their subjects, but they were able to determine blood lead levels on a few of them. These indicated that children in the low-dentine lead group had blood lead levels in the range of 12–37 µg/dL, whereas children in the high-dentine lead group were in the range of 15–54 µg/dL (Rutter, 1980). Because this was a cross-sectional study, data could not be used to show that lead exposure preceded CNS effects. Nevertheless, the study was key in moving the discussion of low-level effects forward. It was the first study of a large group of white working-class children in the general public school population. None of the subjects had any overt symptoms of lead poisoning, yet the effects of lead on classroom performance were statistically significant across the entire range of exposure. In addition, IQ and attention differences were significant between the high- and low-lead–exposed groups (Needleman et al., 1979). Other researchers subsequently found similar effects (Winneke, 1982; Yule, Lansdown, Millar, & Urbanowicz, 1981).

In recommending lower acceptable blood lead levels, the CDC took into account studies showing biochemical effects at low levels of exposure, including "reductions in the biosynthesis of heme (Piomelli, Seaman, Zullow, Curran, and Davidow, 1982), in concentrations of 1,25-dihydroxy vitamin D (Rosen, Chesney, Hamstra, DeLuca, and Mahaffey, 1980; Mahaffey, Rosen, Chesney, Peeler, Smith, and Deluca, 1982) and in the metabolism of erythrocyte pyrimidine (Angle and McIntire, 1978; Paglia, Valentine, and Fink, 1977)" (CDC, 1985, p. 3).

Several prospective studies carried out in the late 1980s demonstrated neurobehavioral effects at blood lead levels at least as low as 10 µg/dL (Bellinger, Leviton, Needleman, Waternaux, & Rabinowitz, 1986; Bellinger, Leviton, Rabinowitz, Needleman, & Waternaux, 1986; Bellinger, Leviton, Waternaux, Needleman, & Rabinowitz, 1985, 1987, 1989; Bellinger, Sloman, Leviton, Waternaux, Needleman, & Rabinowitz, 1987; Bellinger et al., 1984; Bornschein et al., 1989; Dietrich, 1987a, 1987b; Dietrich et al., 1986). Thus, in 1991, the CDC again lowered the intervention level from 25 µg/dL to 10 µg/dL and focused on the importance of primary prevention efforts (CDC, 1991).

DEMOGRAPHIC VARIABLES
PREDICTIVE OF BLOOD LEAD LEVELS

Although almost all young children crawl and put things, especially their hands, into their mouths, some children live in more contaminated environments than others, and therefore these normal behaviors result in greater lead exposure and uptake. Data from the Third National Health and Nutrition Examination Survey (NHANES III) and other current studies indicate that the population living in the most contaminated environment and therefore at greatest risk has not changed over the years (Brody et al., 1994). Although average blood lead levels for all groups fell by 60%–88% between NHANES II (1976–1980) and NHANES III (1988–1991), the highest average blood lead levels are still found among poor black children between 1 and 2 years of age living in the inner cities of large metropolitan areas; 36.7% of non-Hispanic black (referred to below as black) children ages 1–5 years living in such areas have blood lead levels of 10 µg/dL or higher as compared to 17% of similarly situated Mexican American children.[1] (The NHANES III

---

[1] Terminology is listed here according to NHANES usage.

sample of non-Hispanic white [referred to below as white] children living in inner cities is so small that the statistics for this group are unstable; 8.1% of white children in the inner cities of smaller cities have blood lead levels of 10 µg/dL or higher [Pirkle et al., 1994] [Table 1].) Inner-city communities have more older dwellings with lead-based paint than do suburbs and most rural areas. As a consequence of housing discrimination, segregated housing patterns, and limited funds, poor black children are the most likely to live in deteriorated housing with flaking lead paint and lead-contaminated dust. Like other poor children, they are also more likely than children from wealthier homes to have a diet deficient in calcium, iron, protein, and/or zinc, deficiencies that increase the absorption of lead and may increase vulnerability to its adverse effects (Mahaffey, 1981; Mahaffey & Michaelson, 1980). They may also be more likely to have empty stomachs, which increases absorption of lead (Rabinowitz, Kopple, & Wetherill, 1980).

Data on blood lead levels for the U.S. population collected from 1988 to 1991 and presented in this chapter come from NHANES III. The survey sample design and data collection methods and procedures are described in detail elsewhere (Brody et al., 1994). Table 2 shows the mean blood lead levels of children ages 1–5 years in the United States by age category. Mean blood lead levels peak at 4.1 µg/dL in 1- to 2-year-olds and fall slowly after age 2. This age peak holds across race/ethnicity categories and for males and females (Table 3). A higher percentage of 1- to 2-year-old children, compared to 3- to 5-year-olds, have blood lead levels at or above 10, 15, 20, and 25 µg/dL within each race/ethnicity group (Table 4), with two exceptions: 0.4% of white 1- to 2- and 3- to 5-year-olds have blood lead levels at or above 25 µg/dL and about 20% of black 1- to 2-year-olds (21.6%) and 3- to 5-year-olds (20.0%) have blood lead levels at or above 10 µg/dL. Various age-dependent behaviors of 1- to 2-year-olds

Table 1.   Percentage of children ages 1–5 years with blood lead levels ≥10 µg/dL by race/ethnicity and urban status: U.S. 1988–1991

Urban status	All[a]	Non-Hispanic white	Non-Hispanic black	Mexican American
Central city, ≥1 million	21.0	6.1[b]	36.7	17.0
Central city, <1 million	16.4	8.1	22.5	9.5
Noncentral city	5.8	5.2	11.2	7.0

From Brody et al. (1994). Blood lead levels in the U.S. population: Phase 1 of the Third National Health and Nutrition Examination Survey (NHANES III, 1988 to 1991). *Journal of the American Medical Association, 272,* 277–283.

[a]All includes race/ethnicity groups not shown separately.

[b]Estimate may be unstable because of small sample size.

Table 2. Weighted geometric means of blood lead in children ages 1–11 years by age category: U.S. 1988–1991

Age (years)	Population estimate[a] (thousands)	Geometric mean (µg/dL)
1–2	7,476	4.1
3–5	11,165	3.4
6–11	21,748	2.5

From Brody et al. (1994). Blood lead levels in the U.S. population: Phase 1 of the Third National Health and Nutrition Examination Survey (NHANES III, 1988 to 1991). *Journal of the American Medical Association, 272,* 277–283.

[a]U.S. Bureau of the Census, Current Populations Survey, 1990.

lead to greater ingestion of lead in a contaminated environment. These children spend a considerable amount of time on the floor and on the ground. They explore the world by putting things into their mouths. In addition, they carry bottles, food, and security blankets outside with them. All of these behaviors are associated with elevated blood lead levels (Cook, Chappell, Hoffman, & Mangione, 1993; Gottlieb & Koehler, 1994).

In children under 6 years of age, the differences in the blood lead levels between girls and boys are very small (confidence limits overlap substantially). Gender differences are greatest in whites between 6 and 11 years of age and smallest among Mexican American children.

Race/ethnicity is an important predictor of blood lead level (Brody et al., 1994). Black children have higher blood lead levels in all age, urban status, income, and educational categories. Racial disparities between blacks and whites are greatest among the poor. The prevalence of children with blood lead levels ≥10 µg/dL is almost 3 times higher among low-income (family income <1.3 times poverty level) black children 1–5 years old than among low-income white children. In the high-income category (family income ≥3 times poverty level), this ratio falls to 1.3:1. The difference by race in percentages of children exceeding various thresholds is greatest at the ≥20 µg/dL threshold. Black 1- to 2-year-olds are 6.75 times as likely to exceed this threshold as whites (5.4% of black children and 0.8% of white children have blood lead levels of 20 µg/dL or greater).

Overall, Mexican American children's blood lead levels are between white and black children's, but Mexican American children ages 6–11 years have lower mean blood lead levels than non-Hispanic whites. Low-income Mexican American children ages 1–5 years have a lower prevalence of blood lead levels of 10 µg/dL or above than white children of the same age and income status (Table 5). Racial disparities are evident at the 10, 15, 20, and 25 µg/dL thresholds. A greater percentage of black than Mexican American or white children exceed each blood lead level (Table 4).

Table 3. Weighted geometric mean blood lead levels and 95% confidence intervals (CIs) for children ages 1–11 by age category, sex, and race/ethnicity: U.S. 1988–1991

Age (years)	Non-Hispanic white			Non-Hispanic black			Mexican American		
	No.	Geometric means[a]	95% CI[a]	No.	Geometric means	95% CI	No.	Geometric means	95% CI
Males									
1–2	156	3.5	3.1–4.1	137	6.3	5.6–7.2	141	4.2	3.3–5.3
3–5	182	2.9	2.6–3.2	185	5.9	5.1–6.8	232	4.0	3.1–5.1
6–11	236	2.4	2.1–2.7	208	4.5	3.9–5.1	323	3.1	2.4–3.9
Females									
1–2	150	3.6	3.0–4.3	144	5.8	5.1–6.5	157	4.8	4.4–5.3
3–5	170	3.0	2.6–3.5	213	5.0	4.5–5.6	275	3.6	3.0–4.5
6–11	224	1.9	1.6–2.2	182	3.8	3.3–4.4	357	2.8	2.4–3.3

From Brody et al. (1994). Blood lead levels in the U.S. population: Phase 1 of the Third National Health and Nutrition Examination Survey (NHANES III, 1988 to 1991). *Journal of the American Medical Association, 272,* 277–283.
[a]Geometric means and 95% CI in µg/dL.

Table 4. Percentage of children ages 1–5 years at or above selected blood lead levels by age category and race/ethnicity: U.S. 1988–1991

	Age (years)	Blood lead levels (%)				
		≥25 µg/dL	≥20 µg/dL	≥15 µg/dL	≥10 µg/dL	≥5 µg/dL
All[a]	1–5	0.5	1.1	2.7	8.9	33.2
Non-Hispanic white	1–2	0.4	0.8	2.1	8.5	34.2
	3–5	0.4	0.4	0.7	3.7	21.3
Non-Hispanic black	1–2	1.4	5.4	10.2	21.6	63.9
	3–5	0.8	2.9	6.0	20.0	54.5
Mexican American	1–2	1.0	1.9	2.9	10.1	41.4
	3–5	0.7	0.7	1.4	6.8	34.5

From Brody et al. (1994). Blood lead levels in the U.S. population: Phase 1 of the Third National Health and Nutrition Examination Survey (NHANES III, 1988 to 1991). *Journal of the American Medical Association, 272*, 277–283.

[a]All includes race/ethnicity groups not shown separately.

Children from low-income families have higher mean blood levels than higher-income children (Table 5). Low-income children (1–5 years old) are more than 3 times as likely to have blood lead levels of 10 µg/dL or greater (16.3%) than middle-income children (4.0%). These differences are much greater for blacks (28.4%) than for other race/ethnic groups (8.9%). The differences between middle- and high-income families are smaller overall and within and across race/ethnicity categories (Table 5) (Brody et al., 1994).

The disparity in blood lead levels by race/ethnicity is highest among poor children living in the central city of large standard metropolitan statistical areas (Table 1). Among these children, there are twice as many black children (36.7%) as Hispanics (17%) who have blood lead levels ≥10 µg/dL. However, urban status does not have a large impact on the percentage of white children with blood lead levels exceeding the 10 µg/dL threshold (6%–8% in central cities compared to 5% outside of central cities). In contrast, the prevalence of elevated blood lead (≥10 µg/dL) is three times lower among black children living outside the central city (11%) as among those living within central cities of large metropolitan areas (36.7%). The percentage of Mexican American children exceeding this threshold is more than twice as great for those living in central cities of large metropolitan areas (17%) as for those living outside the central city (7%).

These data should not be taken to suggest that rural children are always at less risk than urban children. A 1994 study of more than 20,000 mostly low-income children (age 6 months to 5 years) in North Carolina found that both black and white children living in rural counties were at greater risk of exceeding every blood lead level threshold from 10 µg/dL to 45 µg/dL than their urban counterparts. The odds ratios for black race, 2.1 (95% confidence interval = 1.7–2.5) and rural county, 1.9 (95% confidence interval = 1.6–2.4) were essentially equal.

Table 5. Percentage of children ages 1–5 years with blood lead levels ≥10 µg/dL by race and income level: U.S. 1988–1991

Income level[a]	All (%)[b]	Non-Hispanic white (%)	Non-Hispanic black (%)	Mexican American (%)
Low	16.3	9.8	28.4	8.8
Middle	5.4	4.8	8.9	5.6
High	4.0	4.3	5.8	0.0[c]

From Brody et al. (1994). Blood lead levels in the U.S. population: Phase 1 of the Third National Health and Nutrition Examination Survey (NHANES III, 1988 to 1991). *Journal of the American Medical Association, 272,* 277–283.

[a]Income level was defined by poverty/income ratio (PIR) categorized as low (0<PIR<1.30), middle (1.30≤PIR<3.00), and high (PIR≥3.00). Persons with missing information on income are not included in the analysis of income level.

[b]All includes race/ethnicity groups not shown separately.

[c]Estimate may be unstable because of small sample size.

In North Carolina, rural counties have a higher percentage of older housing and a higher percentage of children living in poverty than urban counties. However, this study was limited because it focused on low-income children and because the urban counties included large suburban areas (Norman, Brodley, Hertz-Picciotto, & Newton, 1994).

A study of 4,500 inner-city, suburban, and rural children in and around Washington, D.C., found that although the inner-city children (almost all black and low-income) had the highest mean blood levels (10.4 µg/dL) as might be expected, the children living in rural Maryland and Virginia (race not stated) had blood lead levels slightly higher (4.3 µg/dL) than those living in suburban Maryland (4.2 µg/dL) (almost all white and having private insurance) (Rifai et al., 1993). The percentage of children with blood lead levels ≥10 µg/dL was twice as high in the rural as in the suburban sample (5.8% compared to 2.4%); 18.6% of the inner-city children had blood lead levels greater than or equal to this threshold. This study had only small numbers of rural children.

These data show that it is important to remember that, although demographic factors are useful in targeting intervention activities, they are only markers for such factors as older deteriorated housing and nutritional deficiencies, which actually lead to increased exposure and uptake of lead, and that no community can be assumed to be free from this ubiquitous toxin.

Regressions on the NHANES III data found that lower educational achievement of a child's primary caregiver and living in the Northeast were also significant predictors of higher blood lead levels in children ages 1–5 years. Region was confounded by the fact that blood lead samples were taken in the Northeast and Midwest during the summer and in the South and West during the winter months. Blood lead levels are generally higher during the summer (Brody et al., 1994).

SECULAR TRENDS

Blood lead levels for the entire population and for all demographic subgroups have declined dramatically since the mid-1970s. These trends can be seen clearly by comparing data for black and white children from NHANES II collected between 1976 and 1980 to data from NHANES III collected from 1988 to 1991, and comparing data for Mexican Americans from the Hispanic Health and Nutrition Examination Survey (HHANES) collected from 1982 to 1984 to data from NHANES III. Between NHANES II and NHANES III and between HHANES and NHANES III, geometric mean blood lead levels declined by 10 µg/dL in all age categories and in all race/ethnic groups (Tables 6 and 7). Mean blood lead levels for children 1–5 years old declined by

Table 6. Distribution of blood lead levels for Mexican Americans ages 4–19 years by age category: 1982–1984 [Hispanic Health and Nutrition Examination Survey (HHANES)] and 1988–1991 [Phase 1 of the Third National Health and Nutrition Examination Survey (NHANES III, Phase 1)][a]

Years	No.	Geometric means (µg/dL)	95% Confidence interval	Percentiles (µg/dL)						
				5th	10th	25th	50th	75th	90th	95th
Ages 4–5										
1982–1984	269	10.9	10.3–11.5	5.0	6.0	8.0	11.0	14.0	19.0	23.0
1988–1991	349	3.5	2.8–4.3	<1.0	1.4	2.5	3.8	5.9	8.3	9.9
Ages 6–19										
1982–1984	2331	8.0	7.8–8.2	4.0	6.0	6.0	8.0	11.0	14.0	17.0
1988–1991	1188	2.5	2.0–3.2	<1.0	<1.0	1.6	2.8	4.7	7.4	9.8

From Pirkle et al. (1994). The decline in blood lead levels in the United States: The National Health and Nutrition Examination Surveys (NHANES). *Journal of the American Medical Association, 272,* 284–291.

[a]For each grouping, the geometric means from HHANES and NHANES III phase 1 are statistically different (*p* < .01).

Table 7. Distribution of blood lead levels for persons ages 1–19 years by age category: United States 1976–1980 [Second National Health and Nutrition Examination Survey (NHANES II)] and 1988–1991 [Phase 1 of the Third National Health and Nutrition Examination Survey (NHANES III, Phase 1)][a]

Years	No.	Geometric means (µg/dL)	95% Confidence interval	Percentiles (µg/dL)						
				5th	10th	25th	50th	75th	90th	95th
Ages 1–5										
1976–1980	2271	15.0	14.2–15.8	8.0	9.0	12.0	15.0	19.0	24.0	28.0
1988–1991	2234	3.6	3.3–4.0	1.1	1.5	2.2	3.7	5.9	9.6	12.2
Ages 6–19										
1976–1980	2024	11.7	11.2–12.4	6.0	7.0	9.0	12.0	15.0	19.0	22.0
1988–1991	2963	1.9	1.7–2.2	<1.0	<1.0	1.3	2.1	3.5	5.4	7.4

From Pirkle et al. (1994). The decline in blood lead levels in the United States: The National Health and Nutrition Examination Surveys (NHANES). *Journal of the American Medical Association, 272,* 284–291.

[a] For each grouping, the geometric means from NHANES II and NHANES III phase 1 are statistically different ($p < .01$).

more than 70% across all racial/ethnic groups. Because mean blood lead level is and was higher in black than white children, the actual amount decreased further in black children but the percentage decrease was lower in black children than in white children (i.e., 72% compared to 77%). For children from low-income families living in the central city of metropolitan areas with populations larger than 1 million, the percentage decrease was even lower, only 60%. The disparity between the mean blood lead levels of black and white children has increased.

Between NHANES II and III, the general population's exposure to lead has been greatly reduced by eliminating lead from gasoline and food cans. The population with greater exposure to the remaining reservoirs of lead—namely, lead paint—experienced a smaller improvement in blood lead levels. The data suggest that black children and poor children were absorbing relatively more of the lead in their bodies from paint than from gasoline or food compared to white children or higher-income children.

As a consequence of decreased exposure to lead, NHANES III showed that the number and percentage of children with high blood lead levels decreased during the 1980s. The prevalence of levels ≥10 μg/dL decreased dramatically in all age and race categories (Table 8) (Pirkle et al., 1994). Among white children, the prevalence decreased from 85.5% to 5.5% leaving 1 in 20 white children with an elevated blood lead level. The prevalence among black children fell from virtually all children (97.7%) to 20.6%, leaving 1 in 5 black children with an elevated blood lead level. The prevalence of blood lead levels ≥10 μg/dL among the Mexican American 4- to 5-year-old children fell from 61.5% to 4.9%. Both the prevalence and number of children with greatly elevated blood lead levels have decreased as well (Tables 6 and 7). During NHANES II, 9.3% of children 1–5 years old had blood lead levels ≥25 μg/dL. During NHANES III, this number

Table 8. Prevalence of blood lead levels ≥10 μg/dL in children ages 1–5 during 1976–1980 (NHANES II) and 1988–1991 (NHANES III) by race and age category

	Percent with blood lead levels ≥10 μg/dL				
	All[a]	Non-Hispanic white	Non-Hispanic black	Ages 1–2	Ages 3–5
NHANES II (1976–1980)	88.2	85.0	97.7	88.3	88.1
NHANES II (1988–1991)	8.9	5.5	20.6	7.2	7.3

From Pirkle et al. (1994). The decline in blood lead levels in the United States: The National Health and Nutrition Examination Surveys (NHANES). *Journal of the American Medical Association, 272,* 284–291.

[a]All includes race/ethnicity groups not shown separately.

dropped by more than an order of magnitude to 0.5%, as did the percentage of children with blood lead levels ≥30 mg/dL from 4.1% to 0.4%. The mean blood lead levels for children in the 95th percentile fell from 28 µg/dL to 12.2 µg/dL.

The epidemiologic data demonstrate that there are children with elevated lead levels in virtually every community and every walk of life. However, these children are concentrated among the poor living in inner cities. In terms of public health policy, we know where the problem lies. We know that lead paint is the most significant source of elevated lead levels and lead poisoning. If common sense and experience in the community do not suffice, census data will allow us to identify tract-by-tract where there are children living in pre-1940, pre-1950, and pre-1960 dilapidated housing. Screening should, of course, focus on these children, but primary prevention efforts—safely eliminating the lead paint hazard from these dwellings—must become the focus and priority of public health efforts to reduce lead's pervasive toxic effects. The elimination of lead from gasoline has clearly demonstrated the effectiveness of primary prevention strategies. The remaining questions are political and economic. During a period when low-income people and people of color are under attack, when Aid to Families with Dependent Children, food and housing assistance, targeted educational programs, Medicaid, and all other programs for at-risk children are threatened, can we successfully abate the nation's number one environmental threat to these same children? Programs could be developed in the private sector involving revolving loan funds and/or requirements that lead hazards be abated as a condition of transfer of title of property, but no program will be instituted without an aggressive effort on the part of the health community and the people affected.

REFERENCES

Agency for Toxic Substances and Disease Registry (ATSDR). (1988). *The nature and extent of lead poisoning in children in the United States: A report to Congress* (Doc. No. 992966). Atlanta, GA: U.S. Department of Health and Human Services/Public Health Service,

Alexander, F.W. (1974). The uptake of lead by children in different environments. *Environmental Health Perspectives, 7*, 155–170.

Angle, C.R., & McIntire, M.S. (1978). Low level lead and inhibition of erythrocyte pyrimidine nucleotidase. *Environmental Research, 17*, 296–302.

Baltimore Health Department. (1971, December). Chronology of lead poisoning control: Baltimore 1931–71. *Baltimore Health News*, pp. 34–40.

Bellinger, D., Leviton, A., Needleman, H.L., Waternaux, C., & Rabinowitz, M. (1986). Low-level lead exposure and infant development in the first year. *Neurobehavioral Toxicology and Teratology, 8*, 151–161.

Bellinger, D., Leviton, A., Rabinowitz, M., Needleman, H.L., & Waternaux, C. (1986). Correlates of low-level lead exposure in urban children at 2 years of age. *Pediatrics, 77,* 826–833.

Bellinger, D., Leviton, A., Waternaux, C., Needleman, H., & Rabinowitz, M. (1985). A longitudinal study of the developmental toxicity of low-level lead exposure in the prenatal and early postnatal periods. In T.D. Lekkas (Ed.), *Proceedings of the international conference on heavy metals in the environment* (Vol. 1., pp. 32–34). Edinburgh, Scotland: CEP Consultants, Ltd.

Bellinger, D., Leviton, A., Waternaux, C., Needleman, H.L., & Rabinowitz, M., (1987). Longitudinal analyses of prenatal and postnatal lead exposure and early cognitive development. *New England Journal of Medicine, 316,* 1037–1043.

Bellinger, D., Leviton, A., Waternaux, C., Needleman, H., & Rabinowitz, M. (1989). Low-level lead exposure and early development in socioeconomically advantaged urban infants. In M.A. Smith, L.D. Grant, & A.I. Sors (Eds.), *Lead exposure and child development: An international assessment* (pp. 345–356). Edinburgh, Scotland: Kluwer Academic.

Bellinger, D.C., Needleman, H.L., Leviton, A., Waternaux, C., Rabinowitz, M.B., & Nichols, M.L. (1984). Early sensory-motor development and prenatal exposure to lead. *Neurobehavioral Toxicology and Teratology, 67,* 387–402.

Bellinger, D., Sloman, J., Leviton, A., Waternaux, C., Needleman, H.L., & Rabinowitz, M. (1987). Low-level lead exposure and child development: Assessment at age 5 of a cohort followed from birth. In S.D. Lindberg & T.C. Hutchinson (Eds.), *International conference on heavy metals in the environment* (Vol. 1, pp. 49–53). Endinburgh, Scotland: CEP Consultants, Ltd.

Berney, B.L. (1993). Round and round it goes: The epidemiology of childhood lead poisoning, 1950–1990. *Millbank Quarterly, 71*(1), 3–39.

Blood lead levels—United States, 1988–1991. (1994). *Morbidity and Mortality Weekly Report* (MMWR), *43*(30), 545–548.

Bornschein, R.L., Grote, J., Mitchell, T., Succop, P.A., Dietrich, K.N., Krafft, K.M., & Hammond, P.B. (1989). Effects of prenatal lead exposure on infant size at birth. In M.A. Smith, L.D. Grant, & A.I. Sors (Eds.), *Lead exposure and child development: An international assessment* (pp. 307–319). Edinburgh, Scotland: Kluwer Academic.

Brody, D.J., Pirkle, J.L., Kramer, R.A., Flegal, K.M., Matte, T.D., Gunter, E.W., & Paschal, D.C. (1994). Blood levels in the U.S. population: Phase 1 of the Third National Health and Nutrition Examination Survey (NHANES III, 1988 to 1991). *Journal of the American Medical Association, 272,* 277–283.

Byers, R.K. (1959). Lead poisoning, review of the literature and report on forty-five cases. *Pediatrics, 23,* 585–603.

Centers for Disease Control (CDC). (1985). *Preventing lead poisoning in young children.* Atlanta, GA: Author.

Centers for Disease Control (CDC). (1991). *Preventing lead poisoning in young children.* Atlanta, GA: Author.

Cohen, C.J., Bowers, G.N., & Lepow, M.L. (1973). Epidemiology of lead poisoning. A comparison between urban and rural children. *Journal of the American Medical Association, 226,* 1430–1433.

Cook, M., Chappell, W.R., Hoffman, R.E., & Mangione, E.J. (1993). Assessment of blood lead levels in children in a historic mining and smelting community. *American Journal of Epidemiology, 137*(4), 447–455.

David, O., Clark, J., & Voeller, K. (1972). Lead and hyperactivity. *Lancet*, *2*(783), 900–903.

de la Burde, B., & Choate, M.S., Jr. (1972). Does asymptomatic lead exposure in children have latent sequelae. *Journal of Pediatrics*, *81*, 1088–1091.

de la Burde, B., & Choate, M.S., Jr. (1975). Early asymptomatic lead exposure and development at school age. *Journal of Pediatrics*, *87*, 638–642.

Dietrich, K.N. (1987a). Low-level fetal lead exposure effect on neurobehavioral development in early infancy. *Pediatrics*, *80*, 721–730.

Dietrich, K.N. (1987b). The neurobehavioral effects of early lead exposure. In S.F. Schroeder (Ed.), *Toxic substances and mental retardation—Neurobehavioral toxicology and teratology: No. 8, Monographs of the American Association on Mental Deficiency* (pp. 71–95). Washington, DC: American Association on Mental Deficiency.

Dietrich, K.N., Krafft, K.M., Bornschein, R.L., Hammond, P.B., Berger, O., Succop, B.A., & Bier, M. (1986). Early effects of fetal lead exposure: Neurobehavioral findings at 6 months. *International Journal of Biosocial Research*, *8*, 151–168.

Eidsvold, G., Mustalish, H., & Novick, L. (1974). The New York City Department of Health: Lessons in lead poisoning control program. *American Journal of Public Health*, *64*, 956–962.

Gottlieb, K., & Koehler, J.R. (1994). Blood lead levels in children from lower socioeconomic communities in Denver, Colorado. *Archives of Environmental Health*, *49*(4), 260–266.

Hernberg, S., & Nikkanen, J. (1970). Enzyme inhibition by lead under normal urban conditions. *Lancet*, *1*, 63–64.

Hernberg, S., Nikkanen, J., Mellen, G., & Lilius, H. (1970). Delta-amino-levulinic acid dehydratase as a measure of lead exposure. *Archives of Environmental Health*, *21*, 140–145.

King, B.G. (1971). Maximum daily intake of lead without excessive body lead-burden in children. *American Journal of Diseases of Children*, *122*, 337–340.

King, B.G., Schaplowsky, A.F., & McCabe, E.B. (1972). Occupational health and child lead poisoning: Mutual interests and special problems. *American Journal of Public Health*, *62*, 1056–1059.

Kotok, D., Kotok, R., & Heriot, J.T. (1977). Cognitive evaluation of children with elevated blood lead levels. *American Journal of Diseases of Children*, *131*(7), 791–793.

Lead-Based Paint Poisoning Prevention Act of 1971, PL 91-695. (Jan. 13, 1971). Title 42, U.S.C. §§ 4801 et seq.: *U.S. Statutes at Large*, *84*, 2078–2080.

Lead-based paint poisoning in children: Statement of the Surgeon General. Washington, DC: U.S. Department of Health, Education and Welfare (USDHEW) (1971), November 8.

Lin-Fu, J.S. (1970). Screening for lead poisoning. *Pediatrics*, *45*, 720–721.

Lin-Fu, J.S. (1972). Undue absorption of lead among children—a new look at an old problem. *New England Journal of Medicine*, *286*, 702–710.

Lin-Fu, J.S. (1973). Vulnerability of children to lead exposure and toxicity. *New England Journal of Medicine*, *289*, 1229–1233, 1289–1293.

Lin-Fu, J.S. (1979). Lead poisoning in children. What price shall we pay? *Children Today*, *8*, 9–13, 36.

Lin-Fu, J.S. (1980). Lead poisoning and undue lead exposure in children: History and current status. In H.L. Needleman (Ed.), *Low level lead exposures: The clinical implications of current research* (pp. 5–16). New York: Raven Press.

Lin-Fu, J.S. (1982). Children and lead—new findings and concerns [editorial]. *New England Journal of Medicine, 307,* 615–617.

Lin-Fu, J.S. (1985). Historical perspective on health effects of lead. In K.R. Mahaffey (Ed.), *Dietary and environmental lead: Human health effects.* Amsterdam: Elsevier.

Mack, R.B. (1973). Lead in history. *Clinical Toxicology Bulletin, 3,* 37–44.

Mahaffey, K.R. (1981). Nutritional factors in lead poisoning. *Nutrition Review, 39*(10), 353–362.

Mahaffey, K.R., & Michaelson, I.A. (1980). The interaction between lead and nutrition. In H.L. Needleman (Ed.), *Low level lead exposures. The clinical implications of current research* (pp. 159–200). New York: Raven Press.

Mahaffey, K.R., Rosen, J.F., Chesney, R.W., Peeler, J.T., Smith, C.M., & Deluca, H.F. (1982). Association between age, blood lead concentration, and serum 1,25-dihydroxycholecalciferol levels in children. *American Journal of Clinical Nutrition, 35,* 1327–1331.

Mellins, R.B., & Jenkins, C.D. (1955). Epidemiological and psychological study of lead poisoning in children. *Journal of the American Medical Association, 158*(1), 15–20.

Millar, J.A., Cummings, R.L.C., Battistini, V., Carswell, F., & Goldberg, A. (1970). Lead and delta-amino-levulinic acid dehydratase levels in mentally retarded children and lead-poisoned suckling rats. *Lancet, 2,* 695–698.

Needleman, H.L., Gunnoe, C., Leviton, A., Reed, R., Peresie, H., Maher, C., & Barrett, P. (1979). Deficits in psychologic and classroom performance of children with elevated dentine lead levels. *New England Journal of Medicine, 300,* 689–695.

Norman, E.H., Brodley, W.C., Hertz-Picciottio, I., & Newton, D.A. (1994). Rural–urban blood lead differences in North Carolina children. *Pediatrics, 94,* 59–64.

Paglia, D.E., Valentine, W.N., & Fink, K. (1977). Further observations on erythrocyte pyrimidinenucleotidase deficiency and intracellular accumulation of pyrimidine nucleotides. *Journal of Clinical Investigation, 60,* 1362–1366.

Perino, J., & Ernhart, C.B. (1974). The relation of subclinical lead level to cognitive and sensorimotor impairment in black preschoolers. *Journal of Learning Disorders, 7,* 26–30.

Perlstein, M.A., & Attala, R. (1966). Neurologic sequelae of plumbism in children. *Clinical Pediatrics, 5,* 292–298.

Piomelli, S., Seaman, C., Zullow, D., Curran, A., & Davidow, B. (1982). Threshold for lead damage to heme synthesis in urban children. *Proceedings of the National Academy of Science, 79,* 3335–3339.

Piomelli, S., & Wolff, J.A. (1994). Childhood lead poisoning in the '90's. *Pediatrics, 93,* 508–510.

Pirkle, J.L., Brody, D.J., Gunter, E.W., Kramer, R.A., Paschal, D.C., Flegal, K.M., & Matte, T.D. (1994). The decline in blood lead levels in the United States: The National Health and Nutrition Examination Surveys (NHANES). *Journal of the American Medical Association, 272,* 284–291.

Rabinowitz, M.B., Kopple, J.D., & Wetherill, G.W. (1980). Effect of food intake and fasting on gastrointestinal lead absorption in humans. *American Journal of Clinical Nutrition, 33,* 1784–1788.

Rifai, N., Cohen, G., Wolf, M., Cohen, L., Fraser, C., Savory, J., & DePalma, L. (1993). Incidence of lead poisoning in young children from inner-city, suburban, and rural communities. *Therapeutic Drug Monitoring, 15,* 71–74.

Rosen, J.F., Chesney, R.W., Hamstra, A., DeLuca, H.F., & Mahaffey, K.R. (1980). Reduction in 1,25 dihydroxyvitamin D in children with increased lead absorption. *New England Journal of Medicine, 302,* 1128–1131.

Rummo, J.H. (1974). Intellectual and behavioral effects of lead poisoning in children. Doctoral dissertation, University of North Carolina, Chapel Hill.

Rutter, M. (1980). Raised lead levels and impaired cognitive/behavioral functioning. *Developmental Medicine and Child Neurology, 42*(Suppl.), 1–26.

Sayre, J.W., Charney, E., & Vostal, J. (1974). House and hand dust as a potential source of childhood lead exposure. *American Journal of Diseases of Children, 127,* 167–170.

Secchi, G.C., Erba, L., & Cambiaghi, G. (1974). Delta amino levulinic acid dehydratase activity of erythrocytes and liver tissue in man. Relationship to lead exposure. *Archives of Environmental Health, 28,* 130–132.

Smith, H.D. (1954). Lead poisoning in children. *American Journal of Nursing, 54*(6), 730–738.

U.S. Department of Health, Education and Welfare (USDHEW). (1970, November 8). *Medical aspects of lead poisoning.* Statement of the surgeon general. Washington, DC: Author.

Winneke, G. (1982, September 4). Neurobehavioral and neuropsychological effects of lead (letter). *Lancet, 2*(8297), 550.

Yule, W., Lansdown, R., Millar, I.B., & Urbanowicz, M.A. (1981). The relationship between blood lead concentrations, intelligence and attainment in a school population: A pilot study. *Developmental Medicine and Child Neurology, 23,* 567–576.

3

ETIOLOGY OF
CHILDHOOD LEAD POISONING

Michael W. Shannon

"We've lived in this house all my life; 15 children have been raised here. Why does my child have lead poisoning?" This comment is often heard from parents or landlords who are surprised, if not skeptical, after hearing that a child who lives in their home has been found to have lead intoxication (plumbism). It reflects one of many misconceptions about the etiology of lead poisoning, neglecting the complex interplay that often exists between children and the lead-containing environment that surrounds them (Figure 1).

Despite the dramatic reductions in the blood lead levels of U.S. children that have occurred since the late 1970s, there are still an estimated 1.7 million children who, through their relationship with the environment, have been exposed to toxic quantities of lead, with the resultant risk of adverse health effects to the renal, skeletal, hematopoietic, and neurologic systems. Continued efforts to reduce lead exposure require a general understanding of common environmental sources of lead as well as other factors that can selectively place a child at risk for lead poisoning. This chapter focuses on the origins of childhood lead poisoning in terms of both environmental lead sources and susceptibility factors.

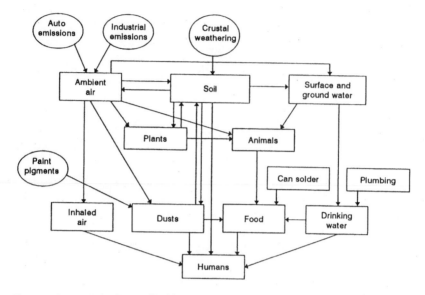

Figure 1. Sources and pathways of lead from environment to humans. (Adapted from U.S. Environmental Protection Agency [1986].)

ENVIRONMENTAL LEAD SOURCES

Air

Worldwide, airborne lead makes the greatest contribution to background blood lead levels, because of both its ubiquity and the efficiency with which lead is absorbed from the respiratory tract. The two major sources of ambient lead contamination are automobile exhausts and industrial emissions.

The addition of tetraethyl lead to gasoline began in 1923 as a means of cheaply increasing the octane activity of less refined fuel. Over the subsequent 50 years, automobile exhausts released more than 30 million tons of lead into the atmosphere. Epidemiologic data have identified a strong correlation between the use of leaded gasoline and blood lead levels (Figure 2). In 1970, the U.S. Congress enacted an amendment (PL 93-15) to the Clean Air Act (PL 88-206), requiring a phaseout of leaded gasoline use (42 U.S.C. § 7545). It is noteworthy that this phaseout was dictated more by the incompatibility of leaded gasoline with catalytic converters than by the desire to reduce population exposures to lead. The elimination of leaded gasoline in the United States was completed in 1995.

The implementation of the Clean Air Act amendment remains one of the most successful public health measures ever instituted. The contribution of lead from gasoline to lead burden has been strikingly illustrated by the fall in blood lead levels that has occurred in the

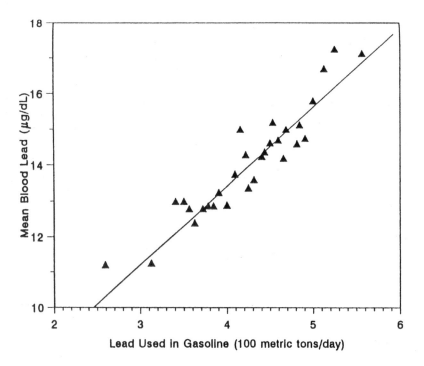

Figure 2. U.S. mean blood lead versus lead used in gasoline. (From Schwartz, J., & Pitcher, H. [1989]. The relationship between gasoline lead and blood lead in the United States. *Official Statistics, 5,* 423; reprinted by permission.)

United Sates in parallel with the diminishing use of lead-containing gasoline (Bushnell & Jaeger, 1986; U.S. Department of Housing and Urban Development, 1990) (Figure 3). The phaseout of leaded gasoline has been credited with reducing blood lead levels in Americans by as much as 60% (Hayes et al., 1994).

Historically, smelters and other industrial sites with a high degree of lead usage have been an important source of atmospheric lead contamination. Although increasingly strict environmental regulations have reduced the degree of environmental pollution, emissions of lead into air and water have produced lead poisoning in entire communities. Many of these areas have now been declared toxic waste sites under the Comprehensive Environmental Response, Compensation, and Liability Act of 1980 (the Superfund Act) (PL 96-510) and are undergoing lead abatement.

In the United States, under present conditions, airborne lead is considered a relatively low-dose source of lead. In other countries, where local economy mandates continued use of leaded gasoline and there is less regulation of industry, lead in the air produces background blood lead levels of 15–20 µg/dL (versus a current background

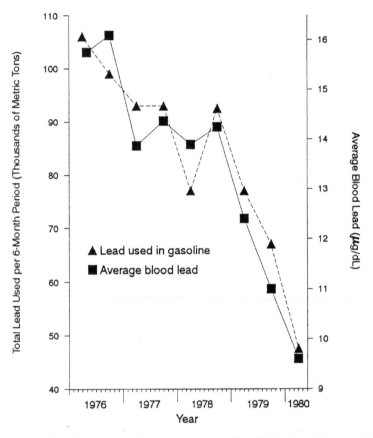

Figure 3.   Lead used in gasoline production and average NHANES II blood lead (February 1976—February 1980). (From Annest, J.L. [1983]. Trends in the blood lead levels of the United States population: The Second National Health and Nutrition Examination Survey [NHANES], 1976–1980. In M. Rutter & R.R. Jones [Eds.], *Lead versus health* [pp. 33–58]. New York: John Wiley & Sons; reprinted by permission.)

lead level in American children of 2.8 µg/dL) (Brody et al., 1994; Orlando et al., 1994).

   Less common sources of airborne lead include improper bridge repair (uncontained paint removal) and the practice of burning battery casings for heat. Occasionally used as a cheap source of heat, discarded lead-based batteries can produce high concentrations of lead vapor when burned, resulting in severe lead intoxication.

Food

Food has not been generally considered a significant source of lead. However, until recently, food was the second largest contributor of background lead to both children and adults.

There are several means by which lead can contaminate food (Table 1). The most important of these mechanisms has been the use of canned foods. Storage cans are constructed by sealing the sheet metal cylinder with a seam of lead solder. With this design, the solder seam comes into direct contact with food, causing lead to leach from the solder. Depending on the pH of the contained food, with those having an acidic pH being the most effective lead solvents, the solder seam may increase the lead content of such canned food by a factor of up to 4,000. The use of lead solder seams in can production was banned in 1991, although cans predating this year are still ubiquitous. Like the phaseout of lead in gasoline, the reduced use of soldered cans has been reflected by marked declines in background lead levels among U.S. citizens.

Another important mechanism by which lead can contaminate food is that of food storage in lead-containing vessels. For example, clay pots often contain galena (lead sulfide), which is easily leached into food or beverage. In addition to lead from clay, decorative glazes may contain bioavailable lead (Acra et al., 1981; Klein et al., 1970). Because of these risks, the Food and Drug Administration (FDA) established standards for maximal concentrations of lead that can be found in kitchenware. These include (measurements performed after an acid wash): plates and other flatware, 3 ppm; cups and mugs, 0.5 ppm; bowls, 2 ppm; pitchers, 0.5 ppm; and large holloware, 1.0 ppm. Surveillance studies have discovered that many popular forms of U.S.-made table china contain quantities of lead that exceed FDA limits. Imported kitchenware, whether bought in a store or imported by immigrant families, is more likely to contain concentrations of lead that exceed federal safety standards (Wilson & Card, 1986).

A third mechanism by which lead can enter the diet is through contamination of home-grown garden vegetables. Lead from either soil or air can fall onto produce, causing surface contamination that will not be removed without diligent cleaning. This is a particular risk for gardens that are placed close to roadways (American Academy of Pedi-

Table 1. Potential sources of lead-contaminated food

Source	Mechanism
Canned foods	Lead solder seam

Storage and cooking vessels
  Clay pots
  Ceramic-glazed dishes
	Leaching of lead into food or beverage

Plates and other kitchenware	Surface contamination by dust (during renovation or deleading)
Home-grown vegetables	Surface contamination or lead incorporation

atrics, 1993). Lead can also be incorporated into the vegetable's flesh. Those green, leafy vegetables that are capable of incorporating iron (e.g., spinach, lettuce, chard, kale) can also incorporate lead if grown in lead-contaminated soil. Root vegetables with leafy green tops (beets, turnips, radishes) also have some capacity to incorporate lead (Camerlynck & Kiekens, 1982).

Water

The potential importance of water as a source of lead poisoning has been recognized for decades; reports of communitywide lead poisoning from the use of lead-contaminated water were once common before control measures were instituted (Beattie, Dagg, Goldberg, Wang, & Ronald, 1972; Beattie, Moore, Devenay, Miller, & Goldberg, 1972).

In the United States, the lead content of water has been placed under regulation of the U.S. Environmental Protection Agency (EPA) through the Safe Drinking Water Act (SDWA, 1974, PL 93-523, 42 U.S.C. §§ 300f–300j-9). In the 1990s, EPA has controlled the lead content of public water supplies by establishing a maximum containment level (MCL) of 50 ppb. In 1991, in an effort to further reduce population exposures to lead from water, the MCL was replaced by an action level of 15 ppb. Under these revised guidelines, source lead control measures must be implemented by the water supplier if lead-contaminated water is found in a substantial number of residential water circuits within a community. An EPA study (EPA, 1993) found that 130 large municipalities throughout the United States provide water that exceeds the action level. These distribution systems serve an estimated 32 million customers in 26 states. A system of lead control measures has been implemented to bring these systems in compliance over the next decade. For example, because lead dissolves more readily in acidic water, pH is a key factor in determining lead concentration. Because so many water sources in the United States have experienced a fall in pH due to acid rain, alkalinization is an essential part of water processing.

From water supply to drinking source, there are a number of points at which water can become contaminated by lead. Even when public water sources have lead concentrations within federal standards, there are a number of subsequent lead sources that can contaminate the water. The composition of the plumbing circuit is the most influential of these sources. Until the 1950s, water pipes were made with lead. Over the last four decades, lead pipes have been replaced by copper pipes, and newer plumbing circuits are constructed with polyvinyl chlorides. However, despite the use of these alternatives, as many as 50% of common and residential plumbing circuits still contain lead pipes. The risk of lead intoxication from these pipes is theoretically reduced by the mineral deposits that eventually form in their lumens, creating a mechanical barrier against the water's direct contact with the pipe.

When lead-containing pipes were replaced with copper pipes, continued lead hazards were produced by the use of lead solder at the pipe joints; the use of lead solder for plumbing was banned by the EPA in 1986. Therefore, all plumbing circuits constructed before 1986 have a high probability of containing lead. Finally, brass, an alloy of copper and zinc that occasionally contains small amounts of lead, may be used in plumbing fixtures and well water pumps. Brass may also contain leachable lead.

Public health investigations of lead-contaminated water have directed considerable attention to the drinking fountains in public schools. Older schools have been found to have fountains that produce water with lead concentrations exceeding 300 ppb. These high lead concentrations result both from the age of the plumbing circuits and from the extended periods for which water remains unmoved within the circuit (e.g., over the weekend).

Infants are particularly vulnerable to lead intoxication from water. In the first 6–9 months of life, those infants who are fed powdered or concentrated formulas that must be reconstituted with water have water intakes averaging 100–150 mL/kg daily. Because of this large volume (on a per weight basis), even low concentrations of lead in water can be sufficient to produce elevated blood lead levels. In the Lead Treatment Program of Children's Hospital, Boston, an investigation into the origins of lead intoxication among infants identified nine who were lead poisoned as a result of lead-contaminated infant formula (Shannon & Graef, 1992) (Table 2). Specific practices that were asso-

Table 2. Cases resulting from formula preparation with lead-contaminated water

Case	Age (mo)	Confirmed	Peak PbB[a] (μg/dL)	Lead source	[Pb] (ppb)
1	4	−	31	Boiled water	
2	4	−	30	Boiled water	
3	9	+	21	Boiled water	142
4	9	+	47	Boiled water	1.0×10^3
5	9	+	41	Boiled water	117
6	9	+	55	Lead vessel	3.5×10^3
7	12	+	48	Lead vessel	1.7×10^3
8	12	+	57	Lead vessel[b]	2.0×10^5
9	12	+	40	Morning water[c]	150

From Shannon, M.W., & Graef, J. (1992). Lead intoxication from lead-contaminated water used to reconstitute infant formula. *Clinical Pediatrics, 28,* 89; reprinted by permission.

[a]PbB, blood lead concentration.

[b]Formula prepared with spring water only.

[c]Previously reported in Shannon and Graef (1989).

ciated with the lead contamination of water were 1) use of first-draw water to make formula (first-draw water having the highest lead concentration of the day), 2) use of hot tap water (which leaches lead more efficiently than cold water), 3) boiling of water in a vessel that contained lead (e.g., an old, imported, lead solder–seamed kettle), and 4) excessive boiling of water (which risks evaporation of free water, thereby increasing the concentration of lead within the water) (Shannon & Graef, 1989, 1992). Severe lead poisoning in young infants as a result of ingesting contaminated water has also been reported by others (Lockitch et al., 1991).

Soil

Airborne lead is eventually deposited on soil, contaminating land surfaces to depths of up to several inches. The soils adjacent to roadways may contain lead concentrations as high as 10,000 ppm; similar concentrations have been found in urban playgrounds. Near lead-emitting industrial operations, the concentration of lead in soil can be 50,000–60,000 ppm. Although soil generally makes little contribution to background blood lead levels at concentrations of 50–200 ppm, it is estimated that each 100-ppm increase in soil lead above 50 ppm adds a 1- to 2-µg/dL increase in blood lead level (American Academy of Pediatrics, 1987).

The mechanisms by which lead-contaminated soil increases a child's lead burden are multiple. First, as a natural part of outdoor play, children get dirty hands, particularly if there is inadequate lawn to cover exposed soil. Normal hand-to-mouth activity (or frank pica) will then result in ingestion of this soil (Sayre, Charney, Vostal, & Pless, 1974). Second, soil can be imported into the home through routine daily activities, becoming a part of interior dust. Finally, lead in soil can contaminate vegetables grown at home.

In 1986, the EPA funded the Three-City Study (Baltimore, Boston, Cincinnati) (Weitzman et al., 1993) in order to determine whether the removal of lead from soil could effect a sustained reduction in the blood lead of children. After interventions that included soil abatement alone as well as soil plus dust (interior and/or exterior) abatement, children were followed longitudinally. Results of the study were mixed. In Boston, mean soil lead reductions of 1,856 ppm produced lead reductions of 0.8–1.6 µg/dL at 11 months postabatement (Weitzman et al., 1993). In Baltimore, soil abatement produced only temporary reductions in blood lead. In Cincinnati, despite abatement of soil as well as *exterior* dust, no sustained reduction in blood lead levels could be achieved. Collectively, these studies confirmed the belief that lead in soil does make a modest contribution to background blood lead levels in children. However, the Three-City Study was unable to clearly demonstrate that abatement of lead from soil would be a successful means of reducing childhood lead exposure. In 1994, largely on the basis of these data, the EPA published national guidelines for the management of lead hazards in soil (Title X, Housing and Community Development Act of 1992, PL 102-550: Section 403 Guidelines). According to these guidelines, soil lead concentrations of <400 ppm require no action. For soil with lead concentrations of 400–5,000 ppm in those areas expected to be used by children, containment measures (e.g., placement of an exposure barrier such as shrubs, grass, or mulch) are recommended. For soil with lead concentrations of >5,000 ppm, soil abatement is recommended regardless of the potential contact by children.

Paint

The widespread addition of lead to paint began in the early 20th century. Added principally in the form of lead carbonate, the metal kept colors vivid and durable. Endowed with these qualities, lead-based paint became most popular in the northeastern United States, where the prevalence of homes containing lead-based paint remains the highest in the country. It is notable that in Canada, where temperature extremes gave greater cause for the use of lead paint, lead was phased out of residential paints early in this century. When it became tragically evident in the 1950s and 1960s that lead paint was the major cause of severe, often fatal childhood lead poisoning, the U.S. Consumer Product Safety Commission enacted regulations in 1977 prohibiting the sale of paints for use on exposed interior or exterior residential surfaces if they contained more than 0.06% lead by weight in the dry, solid form (American Academy of Pediatrics, 1993). Other types of paint (e.g., military, airplane, marine) are exempt from this requirement and continue to contain lead.

Despite the elimination of lead from paint in 1977, decades of use have left as many as 70% of American homes with lead paint. More than 50 million (52%) living units in the United States contain lead paint hazards (Weitzman & Glotzer, 1992). Lead concentrations in paint typically range from 1% to 50% by weight (10,000–500,000 ppm). As this paint deteriorates, it flakes and chips, producing small pieces of concentrated lead that are available to the curious toddler. The vivid color of the paint chip and its notably sweet taste add to the appeal of paint chips to small children. Population sampling has demonstrated that mere presence of lead paint in a home can be directly associated with increased blood lead levels in the children living there in the absence of pica and other at-risk behaviors (Figure 4). When ingested in sizes as small as the fingernail of the fifth finger, a single paint chip can contain enough lead to raise blood lead levels by

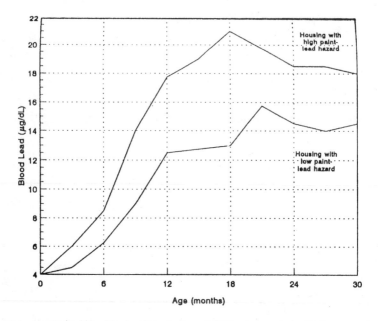

Figure 4. Longitudinal blood lead profiles of groups of children born and raised in housing with and without high-lead paint. Both classes of housing surrounded by lead-contaminated soil and dust. (Data from Clark et al. [1985, 1987].)

more than 10 µg/dL. Repeated ingestion of such paint chips can result in fatal lead poisoning ("Fatal pediatric poisoning," 1991).

In the home, paint chips are most likely to be found in areas that undergo regular mechanical trauma (e.g., door and window frames), on consistently hot surfaces (e.g., radiators), and on the building's exterior (e.g., porches and exterior walls).

Household Renovation and Deleading   When lead-based paint is pulverized to dust, a more toxic form of lead is produced. Lead in dust magnifies the risk of childhood lead poisoning by three distinct mechanisms. First, because absorption of lead from the gastrointestinal tract is inversely proportional to particle size, dust is more efficiently absorbed than larger chips (Chisolm, 1986). Second, an estimated 30%–50% of lead in dust can be absorbed from the pulmonary tract if inhaled (U.S. Environmental Protection Agency, 1986). Finally, even in the child who does not have pica, the combination of dust and normal, age-dependent hand-to-mouth activity will regularly expose the child to large quantities of this "invisible" lead. Current EPA guidelines recommend the following limits on lead concentrations in interior dust: uncarpeted floor, <100 µg/ft²; interior window sills <500 µg/ft²; window wells, <800 µg/ft².

Household renovation activities, including demolition, construction, and paint removal, are all associated with the production of lead dust. These actions often produce lead hazards that did not originally exist by disturbing lead paint that has been covered by latex paint. Because home renovation commonly occurs among middle- to upper-middle-class families, the term "yuppie lead poisoning" has been coined to describe lead poisoning associated with renovation. In cases where the risk of renovation is not appreciated, the family may live in the home during the renovation activities, subjecting all members to lead exposure (Rabinowitz, Leviton, & Bellinger, 1985; Schneitzer, Osborn, Bierman, Mezey, & Kaul, 1990). Parents and other adults who participate in renovation may develop severe lead poisoning (Schneitzer et al., 1990). Domestic pets may also become lead poisoned through renovation activities; their illness may be the first signal of lead hazards in the home (Dowsett & Shannon, 1994). The most hazardous renovation actions are sanding, scraping, and paint stripping with a heat gun (Fischbein et al., 1981) (see also Chapter 9).

Deleading, if improperly performed, can produce lead poisoning, often in children who were not previously exposed (Amitai, Brown, Graef, & Cosgrove, 1991; Amitai et al., 1987; Rey-Alvarez & Menke-Hargrave, 1987). In order to ensure safe removal of lead during deleading, states such as Massachusetts now certify and regulate the deleading industry. In this way, safety measures including temporary alternative housing of all inhabitants, proper protective gear by deleaders, use of chemical strippers rather than heat guns or sanding, confinement of work spaces, scrupulous cleanup, and final reinspection can all be ensured.

Parental Occupations If an adult within the family household has an occupation that is associated with lead exposure, lead-contaminated dust may be inadvertently imported into the home on clothing, shoes, hands, or hair. Lead can be introduced into homes that are otherwise lead-free (Baker et al., 1977). Painters, general contractors, and firearm instructors all risk bringing lead into their homes (in addition to developing plumbism themselves) (Tripathi, Sherertz, Llewellyn, & Armstrong, 1991). The adult who is unaware of this risk may play with a child before changing clothes, thus directly exposing the child to lead.

Congenital/Perinatal Lead Intoxication

A relatively uncommon cause of childhood lead poisoning is in utero exposure (see also Chapter 7). However, lead is efficiently transmitted across the placenta through all stages of gestation. Blood lead levels in the fetus are 80%–90% of maternal blood levels (Ryu, Ziegler, & Fomon, 1978; Timpo, Amin, Casalino, & Yuceoglu, 1979). Lead intoxication is rare in women of childbearing age, occurring only in four groups: 1) those who work in a lead-related industry, 2) those who participate in home renovation activities, 3) artisans who use solder or lead-based ceramic glaze, and 4) women with pica. Lead may be transmitted across breast milk such that women with pre- or postnatal lead intoxication risk exposing their children to lead through their breast-feeding (Rabinowitz, Leviton, & Needleman, 1985).

Lead Intoxication from Mobilization of Preexisting Lead Burdens

Once absorbed, lead kinetics direct it from blood to soft tissues. From here, it is eventually incorporated into the hydroxyapatite crystal of bone, where it is thought to be inert and nontoxic. However, under conditions of increased bone mobilization (Table 3), lead can also become mobilized, producing dramatic increases in blood lead levels. "Recurrent" lead poisoning as a result of bone mobilization has been reported in case series (Goldman, White, Kales, & Hu, 1994; Markowitz & Weinberger, 1990; Shannon, Landy, Anast, & Graef, 1988). Conditions that produce protracted periods in a non–weight-bearing state (e.g., acute paraplegia), have the potential to elevate blood lead levels in previously lead-poisoned children.

Cultural ("Folk") Sources

"Folk" products (i.e., culture-specific traditional materials) can produce lead poisoning in adults and children. These substances are used to treat illness, maintain health, or perpetuate a custom. Many folk products are imported by family members, preventing government agencies such as the FDA from monitoring their safety. Table 4 contains a list of folk medicines known to contain lead.

Therapeutic Agents Two medications originating in Latin American culture, *greta* and *azarcon*, are commonly administered for the treatment of gastroenteritis and other abdominal complaints. These products can contain as much as 90% lead ("Lead poisoning," 1993; Markowitz et al., 1994). Because lead poisoning has abdominal pain as

Table 3. Causes of increased bone mobilization

Zero gravity
Estrogen deficiency
Complete bed rest/acute immobilization
Medications
Corticosteroids
Phenytoin
Phenobarbital
Thyrotoxicosis
Prostaglandins
1,25-OH vitamin D
Parathyroid hormone

Table 4.   Lead-containing cultural ("folk") products

Name	Origin	Uses
Azarcon	Latin America	Laxative
Greta	Latin America	Abdominal pain
Pay-loo-ah	Southeast Asia	Rash, fever
Farouk	Middle East	Teething
Bint Al Zahab	Middle East	Colic
Kohl	India/Africa	Cosmetic
Surma	India/Africa	Cosmetic
Hai Ge Fen	China	Herbal remedy

one of its presenting complaints, a spiral of continued use leads to worsening of lead intoxication.

Cosmetics   *Surma* is a cosmetic widely used in India and Africa; it is applied to the face beginning in the childhood years. Although dermal absorption of lead is negligible, *surma* and similar products can produce lead poisoning through lead absorption across ocular mucous membranes or through lead contamination of the hands, followed by hand-to-mouth activity (Yaish, Niazi, & Soby, 1993).

Other Sources of Lead

Lead-Based Hobbies and Avocations   Adult household members sometimes have lead-associated hobbies or activities that they pursue in the home. (See Table 5 for some examples of other sources of lead.) Examples of this are pottery making, electronic circuit repair, and fishing weight construction (Vance et al., 1990).

Foreign Bodies   Lead-containing foreign bodies can be a source of lead poisoning by many routes. For example, curtain and fishing weights are made in sizes that are easily ingested. Although their large

Table 5.   Miscellaneous lead sources

Lead crystal decanters
Bread wrappings
Crayons
Chalk
Brass water pumps
Newspaper (color print)
Artisan supplies
    Clay
    Paints and glazes
    Solder
Gasoline sniffing (produces organic lead poisoning)
Antique pewter
Calcium supplements (e.g., dolomite)

size generally limits lead absorption, if they are retained in the gastrointestinal tract for extended periods, substantial lead absorption can occur. One report has described fatal lead intoxication in a child who ingested a curtain weight approximately 1 month prior (Hugelmeyer, Moorhead, Horenblas, & Bayer, 1988).

It is unclear whether lead in retained foreign bodies (e.g., bullet fragments) can be absorbed. Although elevated blood lead levels have been found in military troops with retained bullets and shrapnel (Manton, 1994), lead is not absorbed with efficiency from every part of the body (Linden et al., 1982; Selbst, Henretig, Fee, Levy, & Kitts, 1986). The most effective absorption of lead occurs across synovial membranes (Manton & Thal, 1986). There is less persuasive evidence that lead can be absorbed from peritoneal membranes or soft tissues (e.g., muscle, fascia).

RISK (SUSCEPTIBILITY) FACTORS FOR CHILDHOOD LEAD POISONING

Despite the ubiquity of lead in the environment, clearly there are risk factors that selectively place children at risk for lead poisoning while leaving their siblings or playmates unaffected.

Age

Age is perhaps the most important risk factor for lead poisoning. Data from the Third National Health and Nutrition Examination Survey (NHANES III) indicate that blood lead levels are highest between 12 and 36 months of age, diminishing thereafter until the elderly years. There are a number of reasons that this young age group is most susceptible to lead exposure. First, at this age, children master ambulation and become capable of exploring all corners of their environment, finding lead sources previously unavailable to them. Second, toddlers receive relatively less parental attention than infants, providing greater opportunity for unsupervised hazardous behaviors. Third, young children, in exploring their environment, often spend a considerable amount of time at the window, a site that tends to have high concentrations of lead, usually in the form of easily absorbed dust. Fourth, toddlers have not only developmentally appropriate hand-to-mouth activity but also a high rate of pica (i.e., the repeated ingestion of nonfood substances). Fifth, toddlers have a high prevalence of iron deficiency, which increases gastrointestinal absorption of ingested lead (see below). Finally, gastrointestinal absorption of ingested lead is inversely related to age: Although adults absorb only 10%–20% of lead, young children absorb 30%–50%.

There are few epidemiologic data on lead exposure in the first year of life. However, longitudinal data gathered by Bornschein et al. (1987) suggest that important lead exposure begins as early as 6 months of life. Exposure at this young age probably results from early hand-to-mouth activity.

Nutrition

Lead kinetics are strongly influenced by nutrition, particularly iron and calcium balance (Mahaffey, 1990; Mahaffey, Gartside, & Glueck, 1986). Both animal models and human data have proven that diets low in calcium enhance lead absorption. Calcium deficiency not only increases lead absorption but also inhibits lead incorporation into bone. Bone lead levels have been inversely related to calcium intake in population-based studies (Sayre et al., 1974). Iron deficiency is also associated with enhanced gastrointestinal absorption of lead, probably as a result of competition between iron and lead for binding and absorption sites within the small intestine (Barton, Contrad, Harrison, & Nuby, 1978; Markowitz, Rosen, & Bijur, 1990).

Other nutrients have been associated with the development of lead intoxication. A high-fat diet appears to promote lead absorption (American Academy of Pediatrics, 1993). Dietary phytate, found in cereals, decreases lead absorption. Finally, inadequate total calories and infrequent meals (both of which are more likely to be found in children from lower socioeconomic groups) increase the absorption of ingested lead (Sargeant, 1994).

Pica

Pica is the repeated ingestion of nonnutritive substances. Among children, this term is used more broadly to include those who also mouth without ingesting foreign objects and those who bite into objects (e.g., window sills, crib rails). Because exploration of the environment through oral activity can be considered a normal part of child development, the onset of pica is difficult to characterize. However, oral habits begin to diminish after 2–3 years of age; after this, actions that can truly be called pica become more obvious. It has been estimated that 30% of children with pica have lead poisoning (Danford, 1982; Wiley, Henretig, & Selbst, 1992).

Developmental Delay

Children with severe developmental delay, such as autism, have been identified as being at increased risk for lead poisoning (American Academy of Pediatrics, 1993; Cohen, Johnson, & Caparulo, 1976). This risk is most likely accounted for by the higher rate of pica that is found among such children. Also unique among those with severe developmental delay is that oral habits may not spontaneously abate in the second and third year of life as they do in children without developmental delay. As a result, children with significant developmental delay are at risk for both severe lead intoxication and long-term lead exposure.

PATTERNS OF EXPOSURE IN
HIGH- VERSUS LOW-SEVERITY PLUMBISM

In children with lead poisoning (currently defined as a blood lead ≥10 µg/dL), the cornerstone of treatment is to identify the source of lead and to institute measures to reduce or eliminate further absorption. However, the success of this goal is determined by the ability to find a single or point source of lead that can be abated. In children with blood lead levels of 10–20 µg/dL, it is unusual to identify a single source of lead exposure. Instead, elevated blood lead levels represent the sum of exposure to lead from soil, water, food, and dust. Therefore, in children with lead levels in this range, conventional lead inspections that perform only paint analysis may fail to disclose the exact source of lead. In many of these circumstances, there may be little or no lead paint in the home. This finding has brought into question the efficacy of paint abatement alone in reducing blood lead levels and keeping them low in children with levels of 10–20 µg/dL.

As blood lead levels approach and exceed 20 µg/dL, the likelihood of identifying important single sources of lead increases. A detailed environmental history will likely uncover a history of renovation, paint or soil ingestion, unsafe water preparation practices, time spent elsewhere, or some other recognized source of lead. In these cases, removal of the lead source is likely to be highly effective in reducing blood lead levels, occasionally with the assistance of chelation therapy (see also Chapter 8).

Blood lead levels have the potential to include or exclude certain sources of lead, particularly paint chip ingestion. Because lead-based paint chips have such large concentrations of lead (up to 50% by weight), one can generally assume that the child with a blood lead level of ≤20–25 µg/dL has not been ingesting paint chips; children who repeatedly ingest paint chips have much higher blood lead levels.

OBTAINING AN ENVIRONMENTAL HISTORY

In providing intervention for the child with an elevated blood lead level, the initial step is to obtain a detailed environmental history. The

Table 6. Elements of the environmental history

Present residence
General description (age, condition)
Recent renovations
Inspections, deleading
Water or soil analyses, if done
Former residences
Other potential lead exposures
Time spent elsewhere
Lead-based kitchenware
Lead-based "folk" products
Past medical history
Development/milestones
Pica
Witnessed paint chip handling or ingestion
Soil ingestion
Biting into surfaces
Past lead exposures
Occupations/hobbies
Occupations of all adults
Specific practices (e.g., clothes changing)
Work areas in home
Siblings
Ages
Blood lead levels (should be obtained)

environmental history has several components (Table 6). Taking into account all of the recognized etiologies of childhood lead plumbism, these include information about where the child spends time, relevant aspects of the family, social or past medical history, occupations of all resident adults, and blood lead levels of siblings. The goal of the environmental interview (which usually takes 30–45 minutes to obtain) is to develop a complete picture of how that particular child interacts with the environment(s) in a way that readily explains how lead poisoning occurred in him or her rather than a sibling or playmate. It is not until the environmental history is obtained that management of lead poisoning can begin.

SUMMARY

The causes of childhood lead poisoning are multiple and must take into account potential environmental hazards as well as characteristics of the individual child. Once a child is found to have lead intoxication, all of these potential sources must be identified through a detailed environmental history followed by an appropriately directed inspection for lead hazards.

REFERENCES

Acra, A., Raffoul, Z., Dajani, R., & Karahagopian, Y. (1981). Lead glazed pottery: A potential health hazard in the Middle East. *Lancet, 1,* 433–434.
American Academy of Pediatrics, Committee on Environmental Hazards, Committee on Accident and Poison Prevention. (1987). Statement on childhood lead poisoning. *Pediatrics, 79,* 457–465.
American Academy of Pediatrics, Committee on Environmental Health. (1993). Lead poisoning: From screening to primary prevention. *Pediatrics, 92,* 176–183.
Amitai, Y., Brown, M.J., Graef, J.W., & Cosgrove, E. (1991). Residential deleading: Effects on the blood lead levels of lead-poisoned children. *Pediatrics, 88,* 893–897.
Amitai, Y., Graef, J.W., Brown, M.J., Gerstle, R.S., Kahn, N., & Cochrane, P.E. (1987). Hazards of "deleading" homes of children with lead poisoning. *American Journal of Diseases of Children, 141,* 758–760.
Annest, J.L. (1983). Trends in the blood lead levels of the United States population: The Second National Health and Nutrition Survey (NHANES), 1976–1980. In M. Rutter & R.R. Jones (Eds.), *Lead versus health* (pp. 33–58). New York: John Wiley & Sons.
Baker, E.L., Folland, D.S., Taylor, T.A., Frank, M., Peterson, W., Lovejoy, G., Cox, D., Housworth, J., & Landrigan, P.J. (1977). Lead poisoning in children of lead workers—House contamination with industrial dust. *New England Journal of Medicine, 296,* 260–261.
Barton, J.C., Contrad, M.E., Harrison, L., & Nuby, S. (1978). Effects of calcium on the absorption and retention of lead. *Journal of Laboratory and Clinical Medicine, 91,* 366–376.
Beattie, A.D., Dagg, J.H., Goldberg, A., Wang, I., & Ronald, J. (1972). Lead poisoning in rural Scotland. *British Medical Journal, 2,* 488–491.
Beattie, A.D., Moore, M.R., Devenay, W.T., Miller, A.R., & Goldberg, A. (1972). Environmental lead pollution in an urban soft-water area. *British Medical Journal, 2,* 491–493.
Bornschein, R.L., Succop, D.A., Drafft, K.M., Clark, C.S., Peace, B., & Hammond, P.B. (1987). Exterior surface dust lead, interior house dust lead and childhood lead exposure in an urban environment. *Trace Substances and Environmental Health, 20,* 322–332.
Brody, D.J., Pirkle, J.L., Kramer, R.A., Flegal, K.M., Matte, T.D., Gunter, E.W., & Paschal, D.C. (1994). Blood lead levels in the U.S. population: Phase 1 of the Third National Health and Nutrition Examination Survey (NHANES III, 1988 to 1991). *Journal of the American Medical Association, 272,* 277–283.
Bushnell, P.J., & Jaeger, R.J. (1986). Hazards to health from environmental lead exposure: A review of recent literature. *Veterinary and Human Toxicology, 28,* 255–261.
Camerlynck, R., & Kiekens, L. (1982). Speciation of heavy metals in soil based on charge separation. *Plant Soil, 68,* 331–339.
Chisolm, J.J. (1986). Removal of lead paint from old housing: The need for a new approach. *American Journal of Public Health, 76,* 236–237.
Clark, C.S., Bornschein, R.L., Succop, P., Hammond, P.B., Peace, B., Krafft, K., & Dietrich, K. (1987). Pathways to elevated blood lead and their importance

in control stategy development. In S.E. Lindberg & T.C. Hutchinson (Eds.), *International Conference on Heavy Metals in the Environment* (Vol. I, pp. 159–161). Edinburgh, Scotland: CEP Consultants.

Clark, C.S., Bornschein, R.L., Succop, P., Quettel, S.S., Hammond, P.B., & Peace, B. (1985). Condition and type of housing as an indicator of potential environmental lead exposure and pediatric blood lead levels. *Environmental Research, 38*, 46–53.

Clean Air Act, PL 88-206. (December 17, 1963). Title 42, U.S.C. §§ 7401 et seq.: *U.S. Statutes at Large, 77*, 392–401.

Clean Air Act Amendments of 1973, PL 93-15. (April 9, 1973). Title 42, U.S.C. § 7545: *U.S. Statutes at Large, 86*, 11.

Cohen, D.J., Johnson, W.T., & Caparulo, B.K. (1976). Pica and elevated blood lead level in autistic and atypical children. *American Journal of Diseases of Children, 130*, 47–48.

Comprehensive Environmental Response, Compensation, and Liability Act of 1980, PL 96-510. (December 8, 1980). Title 42, U.S.C. §§ 9601 et seq.: *U.S. Statutes at Large, 94*, 2767–2811.

Danford, D.E. (1982). Pica & nutrition. *Annual Review of Nutrition, 2*, 301.

Dowsett, R., & Shannon, M. (1994). Childhood plumbism identified after lead poisoning in domestic pets. *New England Journal of Medicine, 331*, 1661–1662.

Fatal pediatric poisoning from leaded paint—Wisconsin, 1990. (1991). *Morbidity and Mortality Weekly Report (MMWR), 12*, 193–195.

Fischbein, A., Anderson, K.E., Sassa, S., Lilis, R., Kon, S., Sarkozi, L., & Kappas, A. (1981). Lead poisoning from "do-it-yourself" heat guns for removing lead-based paint: Report of two cases. *Environmental Research, 24*, 425–431.

Goldman, R.H., White, R., Kales, S.N., & Hu, H. (1994). Lead poisoning from mobilization of bone stores during thyrotoxicosis. *American Journal of Industrial Medicine, 25*, 417–424.

Hayes, E.B., McElvaine, M.D., Orbach, H.G., Fernandez, A.M., Lyne, S., & Matte, T.D. (1994). Long-term trends in blood lead levels among children in Chicago: Relationship to air lead levels. *Pediatrics, 93*, 195–200.

Housing and Community Development Act of 1992, PL 102-550. (October 28, 1992). Title 42, U.S.C. §§ 1437 et seq.: *U.S. Statutes at Large, 106*, 3672–4097.

Hugelmeyer, C.D., Moorhead, J.C., Horenblas, L., & Bayer, M.J. (1988). Fatal lead encephalopathy following foreign body ingestion: Case report. *Journal of Emergency Medicine, 6*, 397–400.

Klein, M., Namer, R., Harper, E., et al. (1970). Earthenware containers as a source of fatal lead poisoning. *New England Journal of Medicine, 283*, 669–672.

Lead poisoning associated with the use of traditional ethnic remedies—California, 1991–1992. (1993). *Morbidity and Mortality Weekly Report (MMWR), 42*, 521–524.

Linden, M.A., Manton, W.I., Stewart, R.M., Thal, E.R., & Feit, H. (1982). Lead poisoning from retained bullets—Pathogenesis, diagnosis, and management. *Annals of Surgery, 195*, 305–313.

Lockitch, G., Berry, B., Roland, E., Wadsworth, L., Kaikov, Y., & Mirhady, F. (1991). Seizures in a 10-week old infant: Lead poisoning from an unexpected source. *Canadian Medical Association Journal, 145*, 1465–1468.

Mahaffey, K.R. (1990). Environmental lead toxicity: Nutrition as a component of intervention. *Environmental Health Perspectives, 89*, 75–78.

Mahaffey, K.R., Gartside, P.S., & Glueck, C.J. (1986). Blood lead levels and dietary calcium intake in 1- to 11-year-old children: The Second National Health and Nutrition Examination Survey, 1976–1980. *Pediatrics, 78,* 257–262.

Manton, W.I. (1994). Lead poisoning from gunshots: A five century heritage. *Clinical Toxicology, 32,* 387–389.

Manton, W.I, & Thal, E.R. (1986). Lead poisoning from retained missiles: An experimental study. *Annals of Surgery, 204,* 594–599.

Markowitz, S.B., Nunez, C.M., Klitzman, S., Munshi, A.A., Kim, W.S., Eisinger, J., & Landrigan, P.J. (1994). Lead poisoning due to Hai Ge Fen: The porphyrin content of individual erythrocytes. *Journal of the American Medical Association, 271,* 932–934.

Markowitz, M.E., Rosen, J.F., & Bijur, P.E. (1990). Effects of iron deficiency on lead excretion in children with moderate lead intoxication. *Journal of Pediatrics, 116,* 360–364.

Markowitz, M.E., & Weinberger, H.L. (1990). Immobilization-related lead toxicity in previously lead-poisoned children. *Pediatrics, 86,* 455–457.

Orlando, P., Perdelli, F., Gallelli, G., Reggiani, E., Cristina, M.L., & Oberto, C. (1994). Increased blood lead levels in runners training in urban areas. *Archives of Environmental Health, 49,* 200–203.

Rabinowitz, M., Leviton, A., & Bellinger, D. (1985). Home refinishing, lead paint, and infant blood lead levels. *American Journal of Public Health, 75,* 403–404.

Rabinowitz, M., Leviton, A., & Needleman, H. (1985). Lead in milk and infant blood: A dose–response model. *Archives of Environmental Health, 40,* 283–286.

Rey-Alvarez, S., & Menke-Hargrave, T. (1987). Deleading dilemma: Pitfall in the management of childhood lead poisoning. *Pediatrics, 79,* 214–217.

Ryu, J.E., Ziegler, E., & Fomon, S.J. (1978). Maternal lead exposure and blood lead concentration in infancy. *Journal of Pediatrics, 93,* 476–478.

Safe Drinking Water Act of 1974, PL 93-523. (December 16, 1974). Title 42, U.S.C. §§ 300 et seq.: *U.S. Statutes at Large, 88,* 1660–1694.

Sargeant, J.D. (1994). The role of nutrition in the prevention of lead poisoning in children. *Pediatric Annals, 23,* 636–642.

Sayre, J.W., Charney, E., Vostal, J., & Pless, I.B. (1974). House and hand dust as a potential source of childhood lead exposure. *American Journal of Diseases of Children, 127,* 167–170.

Schneitzer, L., Osborn, H.H., Bierman, A., Mezey, A., & Kaul, B. (1990). Lead poisoning in adults from renovation of an older home. *Annals of Emergency Medicine, 19,* 415–420.

Schwartz, J., & Pitcher, H. (1989). The relationship between gasoline lead and blood lead in the United States. *Official Statistics, 5,* 421–431.

Selbst, S.M., Henretig, F., Fee, M.A., Levy, S.E., & Kitts, A.W. (1986). Lead poisoning in a child with a gunshot wound. *Pediatrics, 77,* 413–416.

Shannon, M., & Graef, J.W. (1989). Lead intoxication from lead-contaminated water used to reconstitute infant formula. *Clinical Pediatrics, 28,* 380–382.

Shannon, M., & Graef, J.W. (1992). Lead intoxication in infancy. *Pediatrics, 89,* 87–90.

Shannon, M., Landy, J., Anast, C., & Graef, J. (1988). Recurrent lead poisoning in a child with immobilization osteoporosis. *Veterinary and Human Toxicology, 30,* 586–588.

Timpo, A.E., Amin, J.S., Casalino, M.B., & Yuceoglu, A.M. (1979). Congenital lead intoxication. *Journal of Pediatrics, 94,* 765–767.

Tripathi, R.K., Sherertz, P.C., Llewellyn, G.C., & Armstrong, C.W. (1991). Lead exposure in outdoor firearm instructors. *American Journal of Public Health, 81,* 753–755.

U.S. Department of Housing and Urban Development. (1990). *Comprehensive and workable plan for the abatement of lead-based paint in privately owned housing: A report to Congress.* Washington, DC: Author.

U.S. Environmental Protection Agency. (1986). *Air quality criteria of lead.* 4 vols, Research Triangle Park: U.S. Environmental Protection Agency, Environmental Criteria and Assessment Office. Report Nos. EPA600/8-83/028aF through 028dF.

Vance, M.V., Curry, S.C., Bradley, J.M., Kunkel, D.B., Gerkin, R.D., & Bond, G.R. (1990). Acute lead poisoning in nursing home and psychiatric patients from the ingestion of lead-based ceramic glazes. *Archives of Internal Medicine, 150,* 2085–2092.

Weitzman, M., Aschengrau, A., Bellinger, D., Jones, R., Hamlin, J.S., & Beiser, A. (1993). Lead-contaminated soil abatement and urban children's lead levels. *Journal of the American Medical Association, 269,* 1647–1654.

Weitzman, M., & Glotzer, D. (1992). Lead poisoning. *Pediatrics Review, 13,* 461–468.

Wiley, J.F., Henretig, F.M., & Selbst, S.M. (1992). Blood lead levels in children with foreign bodies. *Pediatrics, 89,* 593–596.

Wilson, T.W., & Card, R.T. (1986). Lead poisoning: Unusual manifestation and unusual source. *Canadian Medical Association Journal, 135,* 773–775.

Yaish, H.M., Niazi, G.A., & Soby, A. (1993). Lead poisoning among Saudi children. *Annals of Saudi Medicine, 13,* 395–401.

4

SCREENING FOR
LEAD POISONING

James G. Linakis
Angela C. Anderson
Siegfried M. Pueschel

Although lead poisoning in children was first reported in the United States at the beginning of this century (Thomas & Blackfan, 1914), it was not until the 1960s that screening programs for lead poisoning were initiated (Lin-Fu, 1992). These initial screening programs, conducted in such cities as Chicago, Baltimore, Boston, and New York, established that many children living in inner cities had high blood lead concentrations.

In 1971, Congress passed the Lead-Based Paint Poisoning Prevention Act (PL 91-695), which represented the first national effort in the United States to identify children with lead poisoning and to clean up sources of lead poisoning in the environment. In the 1980s, federal block grant monies became available to states to develop lead poisoning treatment and prevention programs to include the development of screening strategies. The Lead Contamination Control Act of 1988 (PL 100-572) authorized the Centers for Disease Control and Prevention (CDC) to make grants available to states for the development of comprehensive lead poisoning programs with a focus on the screening of infants and children for elevated blood lead levels ("Implementation," 1992; Lin-Fu, 1992).

In 1991, after new evidence had become available showing that significant adverse neurobehavioral effects may be observed with lead burdens previously believed safe, the CDC established revised guidelines for lead poisoning screening and intervention ("Implementation," 1992). Well-designed studies had become available, indicating that a relationship exists between lead body burden and cognitive function in children. Primarily for this reason, the previously "safe" blood lead level of 25 µg/dL was lowered to 10 µg/dL. The American Academy of Pediatrics (AAP) supported the CDC's new guidelines.

The CDC statement suggested that any burden of blood lead holds the potential for toxic effects as reflected in lowered IQ scores, delayed early cognitive development, and impaired sensory-motor development. Physicians must therefore recognize the significance of the effects of lead poisoning at lower blood levels because impairment of cognitive function may occur at levels as low as 10 µg/dL, even though clinical symptoms are not apparent. In addition, there is evidence that the problem of lead poisoning is not only an inner-city concern but that children who live beyond city limits may be at risk for lead poisoning. Therefore, it was suggested that universal screening of children throughout the United States is the most rational approach to the problem of lead poisoning and that almost all children in the United States must be considered to be at risk.

SCREENING CRITERIA

As recommended by the CDC, a universal screening approach, if carried out appropriately, would have the advantage of identifying all children with lead poisoning ("Implementation," 1992). For a universal screening program to be justified, however, several specific criteria should be met:

The natural history of the disorder must be fairly well understood.
The disorder must be relatively common and detectable in early life.
The disorder must be dangerous or life impairing.
A single design must carry with it a high probability that the disorder is present.
The design must be simple, efficient, reliable, and economical, and at the same time unobjectionable to the patient.
An effective intervention must be available and a therapeutic regimen known that will alter the course of the untreated disorder after diagnosis.
The therapeutic resources must be easily available to the patient, and a medical team must provide long-term follow-up.

Pertaining to lead poisoning screening, it is apparent that most of the above-cited criteria are met. Yet Harvey (1994), who discussed similar concerns, raised a number of questions relating to the seriousness and the prevalence of the disorder, the reliability of test procedures, and the efficacy of intervention.

In addition to the suggested universal screening for lead poisoning, the CDC also recommended that specific questions, which were designed to determine the risk of lead exposure, be asked during children's routine health care visits in private offices and clinics. Physicians are encouraged to routinely ask parents about lead sources in their child's environment. These questions are designed to specify risks but not to replace blood screening tests, because many lead-poisoned children would be missed if the questionnaire alone were used, as detailed below.

There have also been concerns that universal screening would be prohibitively expensive because the major barrier to a universal screening program nationwide is the lack of financial support ("State activities," 1993). Wical (1994) estimated that the cost of the initial screening would be about $440 million. Pantell, Takayama, and Newman (1993) calculated that the *total* cost for screening children would be more than $1.08 billion, or $3,396 per child.

Because of the high cost and for other reasons (Harvey, 1994), some professionals believe that universal screening may not be feasible. It has been suggested that the lower action level for intervention (10 µg/dL) creates unnecessary concern among parents, and questions have been raised among professionals about the necessity of screening all children for these low lead levels. It is argued that such aggressive screening is also inappropriate because effective treatment of children with lower blood lead levels has not been demonstrated. Other opponents of universal screening (Rooney, Hayes, Allen, & Strutt, 1994; Sayre & Ernhard, 1992; Schoen, 1992) believe that the prevalence of elevated blood lead levels is rather low and that the association between low blood lead values and clinically significant neurobehavioral effects is questionable. Harvey (1994) suggested that it would be more efficient to target geographic areas with high-risk children because reliable data on blood lead concentrations in rural children are lacking. Yet in a study reported by Campbell, McConnochie, and Weitzman (1994), it was found that during a lead screening program among high-risk urban children many children were not appropriately screened for the toxic effects of lead. Although many children visited the health center frequently enough to achieve biannual screening, others were not screened and had missed opportunities for lead poisoning screening.

Harvey (1994) also mentioned that a negative consequence of universal screening to the family is the false positives that will result, increasing parental anxieties. A potential disadvantage for society may be a failure to test those children who do not receive health supervision and therefore are at greatest risk. Moreover, new laboratories would have to be developed, new personnel would have to be trained, and the cost of such endeavors would be extensive. Harvey (1994) also contended that, in children with blood lead levels less than 20 μg/dL, there is no evidence that any significant beneficial effect would be achieved through recommended intervention to reduce the blood lead. Chisolm et al. (1994) countered Harvey's arguments against universal screening, documenting that present data support universal screening because

Accurate and reliable tests are available to determine blood lead concentrations
Effective intervention procedures are available
Lead poisoning may have a serious consequence if not remediated

Thus, universal screening for childhood lead poisoning is the desired goal that would permit every child with an increased lead burden to be identified and treated appropriately. Although critical voices are concerned with the high cost of universal screening, the efficacy of intervention, the reliability of the test procedures, and other considerations, the improvement of this aspect of children's health care can be achieved only with the institution of a comprehensive screening strategy.

SCREENING METHODOLOGY

Erythrocyte Protoporphyrin

Until the 1990s, screening for lead poisoning was conducted by measuring erythrocyte protoporphyrin (EP). As explained in Chapter 5, the conversion of protoporphyrin IX to heme is inhibited by lead concentrations as low as 35 μg/dL, resulting in an increased accumulation of protoporphyrin IX, measured as erythrocyte protoporphyrin. There are several laboratory methods for estimating the concentration of protoporphyrin IX. Because nearly 90% of protoporphyrin in erythrocytes exists as zinc protoporphyrin, measures of zinc protoporphyrin by hematofluorometers provide a reasonably good estimate of total protoporphyrin. Other methods measure total protoporphyrin, but, because they first remove zinc from the zinc protoporphyrin, they provide measurement of what is referred to as *free* erythrocyte protoporphyrin ("free" of zinc) (Stanton, Gunter, Parsons, & Field, 1989).

Presently, however, in light of the 1991 revision of the CDC blood lead intervention level from the 1985 level of 25 µg/dL to 10 µg/dL, the EP is no longer considered adequately sensitive to identify the at-risk population. Indeed, the estimated sensitivity of an EP level ≥35 µg/dL for identifying children with elevated blood lead levels was 73% when 1985 CDC guidelines were used (Pb ≥25 µg/dL), but when an elevated Pb was redefined as ≥10 µg/dL the sensitivity was reduced to 26% (McElvaine et al., 1991). Consequently, the blood lead level is currently considered the only acceptable test for screening for childhood lead poisoning.

Blood Lead Concentration

Blood lead concentrations can be measured on capillary blood samples obtained by fingerstick or on venous blood samples. Concern has been expressed that contamination of samples and other difficulties encountered with analyzing capillary specimens may make that method prone to false-positive results or analytical ambiguity (DeSilva & Donnan, 1977; Mitchell, Aldous, & Ryan, 1974). However, venous sampling in infants and small children is frequently impractical, and there is some limited evidence that screening with fingerstick samples may be acceptable when careful attention is paid to skin preparation and avoiding contamination (Schonfeld et al., 1994). Many experts believe that when elevated blood lead concentrations are obtained on capillary specimens, the results should be confirmed on venous samples (CDC, 1991). In those instances where capillary blood samples disclose blood lead concentrations greater than 35–40 µg/dL, it is generally desirable to commence treatment while awaiting the results of confirmatory venous testing.

Analytical Methods for Determination of Blood Lead Concentrations   There are several analytical techniques presently in use for the determination of blood lead concentrations. These are generally variations on atomic absorption spectroscopic techniques (Bannon, Murashchik, Zapf, Farfel, & Chisolm, 1994), potentiometric stripping analysis (Ostapczuk, 1992; Wang & Tian, 1993), and gas chromatography–mass spectrometry (Aggarwal, Kinter, & Herold, 1994), with most laboratories using atomic absorption or potentiometric stripping analysis. These techniques are capable of detection limits approaching 3–5 µg/dL, although this level of proficiency requires careful attention to proper techniques in sample collection, laboratory calibration, specimen handling, and analysis. Blood must be collected using the proper anticoagulant for the method of analysis to be used, and collection tubes must be free from contamination (Crick & Flegal, 1992). Laboratory analysis should include methodology for optimizing the accuracy of blood lead determinations (Jacobson, Lockitch, & Quigley, 1991), and calibration of instrumentation should employ National Institute of Standards and Technology standard solutions and a whole-blood reference panel (SRM 955A, Lead in Blood). In addition, the CDC recommends that laboratories involved in blood lead testing be successful participants in a proficiency testing program administered by a qualified agency such as the Occupational Safety and Health Administration or the program jointly conducted by CDC, the University of Wisconsin, and the Health Resources and Services Administration (CDC, 1991).

Even under the best of circumstances, as noted above, the detection limits of blood lead analytical techniques result in a small amount of analytical variability. As a consequence, a given blood lead value should be considered accurate to within 3–5 µg/dL of the "true" value. Sequential determinations that differ by 2–4 µg/dL are unlikely to be outside of the limit of analytical variance of most laboratories, and therefore such changes should not be considered significant (CDC, 1991). Furthermore, when sequential blood samples from a single individual are analyzed at different laboratories by different analytical methods, the degree of variability is generally increased beyond that of either method alone. Ideally, screening programs should use a single laboratory that employs a single method of blood lead determinations, thereby minimizing differences in levels that might be attributable to laboratory variation.

Radiographic Methods

Long Bone Radiographs   As noted in Chapter 8 on medical management, radiographs of the long bone metaphyses demonstrate growth arrest lines only with blood lead concentrations that are chronically elevated in the range of 50–60 µg/dL or above. Because these levels are considerably beyond currently acceptable concentrations, long bone radiographs are rarely useful in the screening evaluation of a child for lead poisoning.

X-ray Fluorescence   The in vivo measurement of lead in bone by X-ray fluorescence has been under development since the 1970s (Armstrong, Chettle, Scott, Somervaille, & Pendlington, 1992; Gamblin, Gordon, Muir, Chettle, & Webber, 1994; Gerhardsson et al., 1993; Gordon, Chettle, & Webber, 1993; Green et al., 1993; Rosen et al., 1989; Rosen et al., 1991). Although this method is capable of providing a measure of long-term lead dosimetry, it remains largely a research tool (Todd & Chettle, 1994). The potential role, if any, of X-ray fluorescence in screening children at risk for lead poisoning remains to be determined.

In summary, the whole-blood lead concentration represents the standard for screening for lead poisoning in the 1990s. Although this measurement is comparatively easy to accomplish, it is important to recognize that interpretation of the value is subject to several limitations. Blood lead concentrations obtained at a single point in time may be a poor representation of the actual total body burden of lead or of the concentration of lead at the target organs (e.g., brain, kidney, skeletal system). Because a large percentage of an acute dose of lead is rapidly excreted and most of the retained amount is distributed to sites not measured by blood levels, the screening value will be affected by such factors as time from exposure, chronicity of exposure, degree of exposure, and so forth. Thus, when elevated screening blood levels are obtained, further management will be dependent on additional information, such as the degree of elevation of erythrocyte protoporphyrin or measurement of bone X-ray fluorescence (see Chapter 8 on medical management).

CHILDHOOD LEAD SCREENING PROTOCOLS

Background

The 1991 CDC recommendations concerning screening for lead poisoning contend that all children residing in the United States are at risk for lead poisoning. Consequently, the recommendation is made to screen all U.S. children "unless it can be shown that the community in which these children live does not have a childhood lead poisoning problem" (CDC, 1991, p. 39). Communities with homes built before 1960 pose the greatest risk to children because of the common use of paint with comparatively high concentrations of lead through the early 1960s.

Because most children with low-level lead poisoning appear asymptomatic but may still be affected by the subclinical consequences of lead exposure (see Chapters 5 and 6), lead screening is recommended even in the absence of symptoms. Early identification of children with low-level lead poisoning allows for intervention that may prevent those children from later acquiring high lead levels. It also helps target geographic areas where abatement would prevent lead poisoning in other children who subsequently live in those homes and communities.

Age Guidelines

The CDC and the AAP recommend routine screening for lead poisoning in children from ages 6 months to 6 years (American Academy of Pediatrics, Committee on Environmental Health, 1993; CDC, 1991).

These ages were chosen based primarily on a prospective study performed in Cincinnati in which children between 6 and 12 months of age were identified as having the most rapid increases in blood lead concentrations with continued increases up to at least 18 months of age (Clark et al., 1985).

These findings are not surprising, considering that normal hand-to-mouth activity is most common in children in the 6- to 12-month age group and may continue until age 6 years. The elevated rates of increase of blood lead levels between 6 and 18 months also parallel increases in mobility as children learn to sit, crawl, walk, and climb.

Screening of children less than 6 months of age may be indicated for formula-fed infants whose formula has been stored or prepared in lead-containing vessels or prepared with water containing high concentrations of lead (see Chapter 3). Screening also may be required in children older than 6 years who have developmental delays and continued hand-to-mouth activity, as discussed in the section on special considerations.

Initial Assessment

Initial screening of children for lead poisoning should begin at age 6 months with a questionnaire designed to identify children at high risk for lead poisoning. The CDC (1991, p. 43) suggests the following questions:

1. Does your child live in or regularly visit a house with peeling or chipping paint built before 1960? This could include a day care center, preschool, the home of a babysitter or a relative, etc.
2. Does your child live in or regularly visit a house built before 1960 with recent, ongoing, or planned renovation or remodeling?
3. Does your child have a brother or sister, housemate, or playmate being followed up or treated for lead poisoning (that is, blood lead level ≥15 µg/dL)?
4. Does your child live with an adult whose job or hobby involves exposure to lead?
5. Does your child live near an active lead smelter, battery recycling plant, or other industry likely to release lead?

A positive response to one or more questions suggests that the child is at high risk for lead poisoning and should have a blood lead determination at 6 months of age. If the answers to all questions are negative and remain so at follow-up visits, the child is most likely at low risk for lead poisoning, and initial blood lead testing may be performed at 12–15 months of age.

Questionnaires should be modified to target likely sources of lead in various communities (CDC, 1991; Schaffer, Szilagyi, & Weitzman, 1994). For example, in communities where water is a known source of lead exposure or where the use of ceramic pottery is common, questions should be asked that take these factors into account. This is particularly important in regions where the prevalence of lead poisoning is low (Kazal, 1994). Questions regarding lead poisoning should be posed at every well-child visit because potential sources of lead may change (e.g., if the family moves, changes child care locations, begins home renovations).

The CDC questionnaire was found to be an effective screening method when used in a primarily middle-class population in San Francisco where the prevalence of lead poisoning was 6% (Tejeda, 1994). In this study, the questionnaire's sensitivity for detecting children with blood lead levels ≥10 µg/dL was 87%, with a specificity of 75%. The negative predictive value of the questionnaire was 99% (only 1% of children whose guardians answered "no" to all five questions had an elevated blood lead level). A Chicago study, in which the prevalence of venous lead levels ≥10 µg/dL in a suburban practice was 2.1%, also evaluated the CDC questionnaire and reported a sensitivity of 69%, a specificity of 70%, and a negative predictive value of 99% (Binns et al., 1994). This group noted that the sensitivity of the risk assessment questions increased to 83% if the first question was phrased, "Was your house built before 1960?" without any reference to peeling or chipping paint. The authors also suggested that, given the mobility of some patients in their population, a better phrasing of the question might be, "Has your child *ever* lived in a house built before 1960?" This question would capture those children who might have been exposed to lead in a previous home.

Screening Schedule

Because the immature brain is most sensitive to the toxic effects of lead (see Chapter 5), it is important to be vigilant in screening children under 2 years of age. The following screening schedule is adopted from the most recent CDC (1991) and AAP (1993) lead screening recommendations as shown in Table 1 (CDC, 1991; Schaffer & Campbell, 1994).

Screening Schedule for Children Ages 6–36 Months Suspected of Being at Low Risk for Significant Lead Exposure As described above, children found to be at low risk by an initial screening questionnaire should undergo initial blood lead screening at 12–15 months of age. Those with blood lead concentrations ≤10 µg/dL should be tested again at age 2 years. Children with levels between 10 and 19 µg/dL should be screened every 3–4 months until two consecutive measurements are <10 µg/dL, or three consecutive measurements are <15 µg/dL. The child should subsequently be retested in

Table 1.   Schedule for obtaining repeat blood lead levels at various ages, risk levels, and venous lead levels

Age (months)	Risk level	≤10 µg/dL	10–19 µg/dL	≥20 µg/dL
6–36	High	6 mo[a]	3–4 mo[a]	3–4 mo 1–2 mo[b]
6–36	Low	12 mo	3–4 mo[a]	3–4 mo 1–2 mo[b]
37–72	High	12 mo	12 mo	3–4 mo 1–2 mo[b]
37–72	Low	May discontinue[c]		3–4 mo

[a]Switch to annual screening after: two consecutive results <10 µg/dL or three consecutive results ≤15 µg/dL.

[b]Screening every 1–2 months may be necessary during the summer months and in children with moderately high lead levels.

[c]Provided all screenings are <15 µg/dL before age 36 months and no change in environmental conditions.

1 year. As mentioned earlier, blood lead levels should be obtained any time changes occur in the child's environment that may increase lead exposure.

If a confirmed venous blood lead level is ≥20 µg/dL, follow-up levels should be obtained as described for children with lead levels between 10 and 19 µg/dL. However, more frequent screening (e.g., every 1–2 months) may be indicated, particularly during the summer months, when lead acquisition is often the highest; in younger children in whom the effects of lead are the most damaging; and in children with moderately high blood lead levels.

Screening Schedule for Children Ages 6–36 Months Suspected of Being at High Risk for Significant Lead Exposure   If initial questionnaire screening indicates that a child is at high risk for high-dose lead exposure, a blood lead level should be drawn at age 6 months. Children with blood lead levels ≤10 µg/dL should have repeat levels obtained every 6 months until two consecutive levels are ≤10 µg/dL or three consecutive levels are ≤15 µg/dL, as mentioned above. Screening schedules for children with blood lead levels >10 µg/dL are the same as those listed for low-risk children with similar blood lead levels described in the previous section. However, children who also have medical histories that continue to suggest high risk for high-dose lead exposure should continue to have blood lead testing at least every 12 months until age 6 years.

Screening Schedule for Children Ages 36–72 Months   Children between 3 and 6 years of age who have not been tested for lead and are assessed as high risk by questionnaire screening should have a blood lead test performed (see also "Special Considerations" below). These children should then be tested at least once a year until their sixth birthday. Blood lead screening for low-risk children in this age group may be discontinued if all previous screenings indicated blood lead levels ≤15 µg/dL.

Special Considerations

Lead poisoning may be manifested in a variety of ways such as language or developmental delays (see below), hyperactivity, behavioral disorders, abdominal pain, coma and convulsions of unknown etiology, anemia, growth failure, and autism. Therefore, lead poisoning should be considered in the differential diagnosis of children with these disorders.

Children with Developmental Delays   Children with developmental delays and various disabilities may become lead poisoned in a manner similar to children who do not have disabilities and have typical cognitive function. There are numerous children with developmental disabilities who live in environments that create a high risk. In addition, however, these individuals may display behaviors inappropriate for their chronological ages. For example, a child with moderate mental retardation who is 8 years of age may function at a mental age of about 3–4 years. Some of these children with developmental disabilities may also exhibit an increased frequency of pica behavior. This behavior is regarded as pathological if it persists beyond the age of about 18–24 months.

Pica was studied in a cohort of institutionalized persons with mental retardation by McAlpine and Singh (1986). It was found that the prevalence of pathological pica in that group was 9.2%. The occurrence of pica was related to both the degree of mental retardation and the age of the residents. These individuals lived in an environment with high lead content; thus, pica behavior could easily result in lead poisoning. Therefore, all individuals with mental retardation and other developmental disabilities should be screened for lead poisoning, particularly if pica is identified. These individuals may need continued screening beyond age 6 years.

Screening for Iron Deficiency

Because iron deficiency can increase lead absorption from the gastrointestinal tract, children with lead levels ≥ 20 µg/dL should be evaluated for iron deficiency. Iron deficiency may be present even in the absence of anemia; therefore, serum iron, iron binding capacity, and ferritin levels should be obtained to more accurately determine the child's iron status.

Interpretation and Intervention of Screening Values

Currently, blood lead levels <10 μg/dL are considered essentially non-toxic. Levels between 10 and 14 μg/dL suggest low-level lead exposure or acquisition, and follow-up is aimed primarily at early detection of further increases in blood lead levels. Parent education about lead poisoning can be given face-to-face, by pamphlet distribution, or both ways. Blood lead levels between 15 and 19 μg/dL indicate mild lead poisoning and a risk for decrements in neurodevelopmental indices. Parents of children with blood lead levels in this range should receive education about ways to prevent lead absorption and decrease the amount of lead in their child's environment (Kimbrough, LeVois, & Webb, 1994). Children with confirmed blood lead levels ≥20 μg/dL should undergo a medical evaluation and environmental sources of lead should be identified and eliminated.

CONCLUSIONS

Although this chapter provides general guidelines for screening children for lead poisoning, actual practice should be tailored to individual communities and children. Screening questionnaires should include questions that target children potentially exposed to lead sources specific to the community. Furthermore, frequency of follow-up blood lead testing should be modified depending on the child's age and developmental status as well as the known seasonal variations in childhood lead acquisition. Only with an organized, community-based approach to screening can lead poisoning be adequately identified and treated and ultimately prevented and eradicated.

REFERENCES

Aggarwal, S.K., Kinter, M., & Herold, D.A. (1994). Determination of lead in urine and whole blood by stable isotope dilution gas chromatography–mass spectrometry. *Clinical Chemistry, 40*(8), 1494–1502.

American Academy of Pediatrics, Committee on Environmental Health. (1993). Lead poisoning: From screening to primary prevention. *Pediatrics, 92*, 176–183.

Armstrong, R., Chettle, D.R., Scott, M.C., Somervaille, L.J., & Pendlington, M. (1992). Repeated measurements of tibia lead concentrations by in vivo x ray fluorescence in occupational exposure. *British Journal of Industrial Medicine, 49*(1), 14–16.

Bannon, D.I., Murashchik, C., Zapf, C.R., Farfel, M.R., & Chisolm, J.J., Jr. (1994). Graphite furnace atomic absorption spectroscopic measurement of blood lead in matrix-matched standards. *Clinical Chemistry, 40*(9), 1730–1734.

Binns, H., LeBailly, S., Poncher, J., Kinsella, R., & Saunders, S. (1994). Is there lead in the suburbs? Risk assessment in Chicago suburban pediatric practices. *Pediatrics, 93*(2), 164–170.

Campbell, J., McConnochie, K., & Weitzman, M. (1994). Lead screening among high-risk urban children. *Archives of Pediatrics and Adolescent Medicine, 148,* 688–693.

Centers for Disease Control (CDC). (1991). *Preventing lead poisoning in young children: A statement by the Centers for Disease Control.* Atlanta: U.S. Department of Health and Human Services, Public Health Service.

Chisolm, J., Goldstein, G., Cory-Slechta, D., Landrigan, P., Mushak, P., Needleman, H., Rice, D., Rosen, J., & Silbergeld, E. (1994). Lead debate goes on [letter]. *Pediatrics, 94,* 408–410.

Clark, C., Bornschein, R., Succop, P., Que Hee, S., Hammond, P., & Peace, B. (1985). Condition and type of housing as an indicator of potential environmental lead exposure and pediatric blood lead levels. *Environmental Research, 38,* 46–53.

Crick, J., & Flegal, A.R. (1992). Contaminant lead in blood-collection tubes for trace-element studies [letter]. *Clinical Chemistry, 38*(4), 600–601.

DeSilva, P., & Donnan, M. (1977). Petrol venders, capillary blood lead levels, and contamination. *Medical Journal of Australia, 1,* 794–795.

Gamblin, C., Gordon, C.L., Muir, D.C., Chettle, D.R., & Webber, C.E. (1994). In vivo measurements of bone lead content in residents of southern Ontario. *Applied Radiation & Isotopes, 45*(10), 1035–1038.

Gerhardsson, L., Attewell, R., Chettle, D.R., Englyst, V., Lundstrom, N.G., Nordberg, G.F., Nyhlin, H., Scott, M.C., & Todd, A.C. (1993). In vivo measurements of lead in bone in long-term exposed lead smelter workers. *Archives of Environmental Health, 48*(3), 147–156.

Gordon, C.L., Chettle, D.R., & Webber, C.E. (1993). An improved instrument for the in vivo detection of lead in bone. *British Journal of Industrial Medicine, 50*(7), 637–641.

Green, S., Bradley, D.A., Roels, H.A., Mountford, P.J., Morgan, W.D., Chettle, D.R., Konings, J.F., Palethorpe, J.E., Mearman, D.H., & Lauwerys, R.R. (1993). Development and calibration of an in vivo bone lead measurement system, and its application to an industrially exposed population. *Basic Life Sciences, 60,* 295–298.

Harvey, B. (1994). Should blood lead screening recommendations be revised? *Pediatrics, 93,* 201–204.

Implementation of the Lead Contamination Control Act of 1988. (1992). *Morbidity and Mortality Weekly Report, 41,* 288–290.

Jacobson, B.E., Lockitch, G., & Quigley, G. (1991). Improved sample preparation for accurate determination of low concentrations of lead in whole blood by graphite furnace analysis. *Clinical Chemistry, 37*(4), 515–519.

Kazal, L. (1994). Lead questionnaire not always efficient [letter]. *Pediatrics, 93*(2), 192–194.

Kimbrough, R., LeVois, M., & Webb, D. (1994). Management of children with slightly elevated blood lead levels. *Pediatrics, 93*(2), 188–191.

Lead-Based Paint Poisoning Prevention Act of 1971, PL 91-695. (January 13, 1971). Title 42, U.S.C. §§ 4801 et seq.: *U.S. Statutes at Large, 84,* 2078–2080.

Lead Contamination Control Act of 1988, PL 100-572. (October 31, 1988). Title 42, U.S.C. §§ 201 et seq.: *U.S. Statutes at Large, 102,* 2884–2889.

Lin-Fu, J.S. (1992). Modern history of lead poisoning: A century of discovery and rediscovery. In H. Needleman (Ed.), *Human lead exposure* (pp. 23–43). Ann Arbor, MI: CRC Press.

McAlpine, C., & Singh, N. (1986). Pica in institutionalized mentally retarded persons. *Journal of Mental Deficiency Research, 30,* 171–178.

McElvaine, M., Orbach, H., Binder, S., Blanksma, L., Maes, E., & Krieg, R. (1991). Evaluation of the erythrocyte protoporphyrin test as a screen for elevated blood lead levels. *Journal of Pediatrics, 119,* 548–550.

Mitchell, D., Aldous, K., & Ryan, F. (1974). Mass screening for lead poisoning: Capillary blood sampling and automated Delves-cup atomic-absorption analysis. *New York State Journal of Medicine, 74,* 1599–1603.

Ostapczuk, P. (1992). Direct determination of cadmium and lead in whole blood by potentiometric stripping analysis. *Clinical Chemistry, 38*(10), 1995–2001.

Pantell, R., Takayama, J., & Newman, T. (1993). Cost and benefits of lead poisoning screening [letter]. *Journal of the American Medical Association, 270,* 2054–2055.

Rooney, B., Hayes, E., Allen, B., & Strutt, P. (1994). Development of a screening tool for prediction of children at risk for lead poisoning in a midwestern clinical setting. *Pediatrics, 93,* 183–187.

Rosen, J.F., Markowitz, M.E., Bijur, P.E., Jenks, S.T., Wielopolski, L., Kalef-Ezra, J.A., & Slatkin, D.N. (1989). L-line x-ray fluorescence of cortical bone lead compared with $CaNa_2EDTA$ test in lead-toxic children: Public health implications. *Proceedings of the National Academy of Science USA, 86,* 685–689.

Rosen, J.F., Markowitz, M.E., Bijur, P.E., Jenks, S.T., Wielopolski, L., Kalef-Ezra, J.A., & Slatkin, D.N. (1991). Sequential measurements of bone lead content by L x-ray fluorescence in $CaNa_2EDTA$-treated lead-toxic children. *Environmental Health Perspectives, 93,* 271–277.

Sayre, J., & Ernhard, C. (1992). Control of lead exposure in childhood. Are we doing it correctly? *American Journal of Diseases of Children, 146,* 1275–1278.

Schaffer, S., & Campbell, J. (1994). The new CDC and AAP lead poisoning prevention recommendations: Consensus versus controversy. *Pediatric Annals, 23*(11), 592–599.

Schaffer, S., Szilagyi, P., & Weitzman, M. (1994). Lead poisoning risk determination in an urban population through the use of a standardized questionnaire. *Pediatrics, 93*(2), 159–163.

Schoen, E. (1992). Lead toxicity in the 21st century: Will we still be treating it? *Pediatrics, 90,* 481–482.

Schonfeld, D., Cullen, M., Rainey, P., Berg, A., Brown, D., Hogan, J., Turk, D., Rude, C., & Cicchetti, D. (1994). Screening for lead poisoning in an urban pediatric clinic using samples obtained by fingerstick. *Pediatrics, 94*(2), 174–179.

Stanton, N., Gunter, E., Parsons, P., & Field, P. (1989). Empirically determined lead-poisoning screening cutoff for the protoflour-Z hematofluorometer. *Clinical Chemistry, 35,* 2104–2107.

State activities for prevention of lead poisoning among children—United States, 1992. (1993). *Morbidity and Mortality Weekly Report, 42*(9), 165, 171–172.

Tejeda, D. (1994). Do questions about lead exposure predict elevated lead levels? *Pediatrics, 93*(2), 192–194.

Thomas, H., & Blackfan, K. (1914). Recurrent meningitis due to lead in a child of five years. *American Journal of Diseases of Children, 8,* 377.

Todd, A.C., & Chettle, D.R. (1994). In vivo X-ray fluorescence of lead in bone: Review and current issues. *Environmental Health Perspectives, 102*(2), 172–177.

Wang, J., & Tian, B. (1993). Mercury-free disposable lead sensors based on potentiometric stripping analysis at gold-coated screen-printed electrodes. *Analytical Chemistry, 65*(11), 1529–1532.

Wical, B. (1994). Lead: Who bears the burden? [comment]. *Archives of Pediatric and Adolescent Medicine, 148,* 760–761.

5

PATHOPHYSIOLOGY
OF LEAD POISONING

Angela C. Anderson
Siegfried M. Pueschel
James G. Linakis

L ead is a heavy metal with an atomic weight of 207.12 and a specific gravity of 11.34. Inorganic lead salts are primarily responsible for lead poisoning in children. Lead chromate and lead acetate are the lead compounds most commonly encountered in paint. The toxicity of a particular lead compound depends on its solubility in body fluids and its particle size. Lead acetate is highly soluble and is consequently very toxic when ingested. Although this form of lead constitutes a significant hazard in the orally inclined toddler, it does not form dusts readily and is therefore appealing in the industrial workplace because of its low pulmonary absorption potential (Finkel, Hamilton, & Hardy, 1983). Gasoline is a common source of organic lead. Although lead poisoning from gasoline is rare in the pediatric age group, teenage and adult activities such as siphoning and "gasoline huffing" are potentially more dangerous than lead paint ingestion because organic lead is more fat soluble and readily crosses the blood–brain barrier.

ABSORPTION

Gastrointestinal Tract

The primary site of lead absorption in children is the gastrointestinal tract. Although adults absorb approximately 10% of an ingested lead load, children absorb up to 50% of dietary lead. This difference in the degree of absorption is thought to be secondary to differences in gastrointestinal maturation (McCabe, 1979). Most gastrointestinal lead absorption occurs in the duodenum by passive and active transport; however, absorption can occur in all sites in the small intestine (Regan, 1983). There is no feedback mechanism inhibiting the absorption of lead. Approximately 30% of an ingested lead load is retained in the body. A positive lead balance, manifested by increasing blood lead levels, occurs when the daily ingestion of lead exceeds 5 μg/kg body weight (Graef, 1992).

Various dietary factors influence gastrointestinal lead absorption. Lead absorption is better in the presence of liquids than with solids, although absorption is best when the stomach is empty (Goyer, 1993). Deficiencies in trace minerals, particularly calcium, iron, and zinc, also enhance uptake of lead from the gut. For example, iron-deficient rats absorb six times more lead than controls (Regan, 1983). A low-mineral, high-fat diet can increase lead absorption by 50-fold (Barltrop & Meek, 1979). Conversely, the presence of adequate amounts of essential minerals may competitively inhibit lead absorption in the gut. Furthermore, dietary fiber may facilitate lead elimination (Miller, Massaro, & Massaro, 1990).

Lungs

Absorption of lead through the respiratory tract is rapid and efficient. The degree of absorption is dependent on the particle size and the chemical composition of lead. Up to 70% of an inhaled dose of lead is absorbed if the particle size is less than 1 μm (Ellenhorn & Barceloux, 1988). Approximately 90% of lead in gasoline from inhaled motor exhaust is absorbed (Morrow, Beiter, Amato, & Gibb, 1980).

Lead that reaches the alveoli is rapidly taken up by endocytosis (Morrow et al., 1980). Unlike ingested lead, which undergoes first-pass elimination through the liver, inhaled lead passes directly into the circulation. Larger particles that are unable to reach the alveoli can be trapped in mucous secretions, transported by ciliary action to the posterior pharynx, and subsequently swallowed (Barltrop & Meek, 1979). Small particles of lead paint dust commonly found inside window casings and released with repeated window openings and closings are an important source of lead exposure in children.

Skin

Dermal absorption of inorganic lead is negligible. However, tetraethyl lead, an organic form of lead previously used as an antiknock agent in gasoline, is readily absorbed through the skin (Rosenstock & Cullen,

1986). An unusual case of lead poisoning acquired through absorption of a theatrical grease paint that contained 40% lead oxide was also reported (Finkel et al., 1983).

DISTRIBUTION

Once absorbed, lead is distributed into three compartments in the body: blood, soft tissue, and bone. Lead is initially taken into the circulation. Up to 99% of lead carried in the bloodstream is bound to erythrocyte membranes and is nondiffusible. About half of the lead in the red cells is bound to hemoglobin A_2 (Chisolm et al., 1991). Lead can also bind to fetal hemoglobin and does so with an even higher affinity than to adult hemoglobin. Approximately 1%–10% of circulating lead is bound to microligands in the plasma. It is this pool that is capable of crossing cell membranes and therefore can become biologically active (Finkel et al., 1983). Circulating lead has an elimination half-life of 35 days (Ellenhorn & Barceloux, 1988).

Whereas some lead is excreted in feces and urine, significant amounts of circulating lead can become distributed into soft tissue and bone if lead intake exceeds lead excretion. Under steady-state conditions, 5%–10% of lead can be found in blood, 10%–20% in soft tissue, and up to 90% in bone (Graef, 1992). The elimination half-life of lead in soft tissue is approximately 40 days (Kaminsky, Klein, & Duc, 1993; Mushak, 1993; Weeden, 1992).

The half-life of lead stored in bone varies with the type of bone involved. Lead deposited in spongy or trabecular bone, as found in the pelvis, ribs, and temporal area of the skull, is relatively easily mobilized and has a half-life of 3–5 years (Finkel et al., 1983; Mushak, 1993; Rabinowitz, 1991; Weeden, 1992). Lead stored in cortical bone, as located in the midtibia and midfemur, is far less accessible and carries a half-life of approximately 30 years. The periosteum provides another depot for storage and can release lead readily. This site is particularly important in the growing infant in whom larger amounts of this type of bone are found. The toxicokinetics of this compartment have not been well investigated.

ELIMINATION

Approximately 60% of absorbed lead is excreted almost immediately. The kidney provides the primary mode of excretion and is responsible for approximately 60% of daily lead losses (Chisolm et al., 1991). Lead undergoes glomerular filtration unchanged; however, some active transport occurs at high lead levels (Ellenhorn & Barceloux, 1988). Urinary lead concentrations parallel plasma lead concentrations (Kaminsky et al., 1993). The rate of excretion depends on the glomerular filtration rate and renal plasma flow. One must keep in mind that a low urinary lead excretion may not represent a low body lead burden, because plasma lead levels will fall as bony uptake of lead increases.

About 30% of excreted lead is lost in the feces and reflects the amount of ingested lead that is not absorbed plus the amount excreted by the biliary tract (Chisolm et al., 1991; Kaminsky et al., 1993). Approximately 10% of the body's lead losses result from hair and nail growth and from sweat loss.

ORGAN SYSTEM EFFECTS AND THE CLINICAL PRESENTATION OF LEAD POISONING

The majority of children with low-level lead toxicity appear asymptomatic and are discovered on routine lead screening. Occasionally, hyperactivity or developmental delay will incite the clinician to investigate the possibility of lead poisoning. However, despite its often insidious presentation, low-level lead poisoning can cause cognitive abnormalities that may surface when the child reaches school age. The more severe symptoms of lead poisoning (encephalopathy, seizures, colic) are usually reserved for patients with lead levels of 70 µg/dL or greater (see Chapter 6).

There are many factors that place small children at higher risk for lead poisoning than adults:

1. The immature brain of children is more susceptible to the toxic effects of lead.
2. Young children have an increased tendency to ingest nonfood items.
3. Children absorb ingested lead at a rate five times greater than adults.
4. Children in low-income families often have dietary iron and calcium deficiencies that increase lead absorption from the gut.

Lead has multisystem influences with effects on hematopoiesis, central and peripheral nervous systems development and function, hepatic and renal metabolism and performance, and cardiac function. The severity of the clinical manifestations of lead poisoning is related to the duration and intensity of exposure (Biddle, 1982).

LEAD AND HEME BIOSYNTHESIS

Many of the clinical manifestations of lead poisoning are thought to result from the effects of lead on heme biosynthesis. Although heme is primarily synthesized in erythroid precursors in bone marrow and the liver, heme formation occurs in virtually all tissues (Beck, 1981). Lead interferes with heme biosynthesis mainly by depressing the activity of primarily three enzymes in the heme biosynthetic pathway: δ-aminolevulinate dehydrogenase (ALA-D), coproporphyrinogen oxidase (CPG-O), and ferrochelatase (Lubran, 1980; McColl & Goldberg, 1980). Lead blocks the active sites on these enzymes by binding to sulfhydryl groups (-SH) (Beritic, 1981; Goering, 1993; Hermes-Lima, Pereira, & Bechara, 1991; McColl & Goldberg, 1980).

Step 1 of heme biosynthesis involves the condensation of glycine and succinyl coenzyme A to form δ-aminolevulinic acid (ALA) (Figure 1). This reaction is catalyzed by the enzyme 5-aminolevulinate synthetase (ALA-S) and its cofactor pyridoxal phosphate (Beck, 1981;

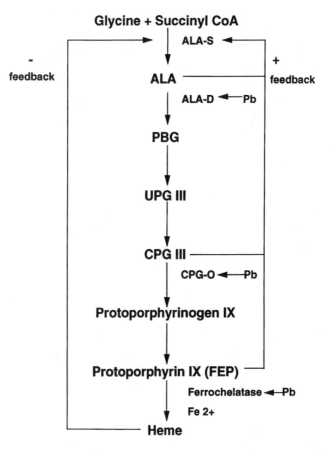

Figure 1.   Effects of lead (Pb) on heme biosynthesis. ALA-S, 5-aminolevulinate synthetase; ALA-D, δ-aminolevulinate dehydrogenase; PBG, porphobilinogen; UPG, uroporphyrinogen; CPG, coproporphyrinogen; CPG-O, coproporphyrinogen oxidase; FEP, free erythrocyte protoporphyrin III.

Lubran, 1980). ALA-S is an inducible enzyme that is normally present in low concentrations in the mitochondria and is the rate-limiting enzyme of heme biosynthesis. ALA-S activity is inhibited by heme production via the mechanism of negative feedback and stimulated by porphyrin accumulation (Lubran, 1980). By inhibiting three enzymes in the heme biosynthesis pathway, lead interferes with heme synthesis and increases porphyrin accumulation, thereby stimulating ALA-S activity in lead-poisoned patients.

In Step 2 of heme biosynthesis, the enzyme ALA-D catalyzes the condensation of two molecules of ALA to form porphobilinogen (PBG). ALA-D is the biosynthetic enzyme most sensitive to lead (Kaminsky et al., 1993). Its activity is inhibited at lead levels as low as 10 µg/dL (Otto, Benignus, Muller, & Barton, 1981). Depressed ALA-D activity results in the accumulation of ALA in the blood and an increase in urinary ALA excretion. Blood and urinary ALA relationships are linear at blood lead concentrations below 3 µM/L and ALA concentrations below 4 µM/L. However, above these concentrations, blood ALA levels plateau as urinary concentrations begin to rise rapidly. A decrease in tubular reabsorption of ALA is thought to be responsible for this phenomenon (Meredith, Moore, Campbell, Thompson, & Goldberg, 1978).

In Step 3, four molecules of PBG condense to form uroporphyrinogen III (UPG III). UPG III then undergoes decarboxylation to yield coproporphyrinogen III (CPG III) (Step 4). The enzymes in Steps 3 and 4 do not appear to be affected by lead (Goering, 1993).

In Step 5, the enzyme CPG-O catalyzes the oxidative decarboxylation of CPG III to form protoporphyrinogen IX. Lead interferes with CPG-O resulting in an increase in urinary CPG III excretion (greater than 0.5 mg/L). In Step 6, the enzyme protoporphyrinogen oxidase stimulates the conversion of protoporphyrinogen IX to protoporphyrin IX.

Iron (Fe^{2+}) is inserted into protoporphyrin IX to form heme in the final step of heme biosynthesis. This reaction occurs in the mitochondria and is catalyzed by the enzyme ferrochelatase. Lead inhibits the activity of ferrochelatase and interferes with the transport of iron within the mitochondria. Consequently, red cells of children with lead poisoning have elevated concentrations of protoporphyrin IX, commonly referred to as free erythrocyte protoporphyrin (FEP) (Goering, 1993). Because lead inhibits the delivery of iron to ferrochelatase, zinc is substituted into protoporphyrin in its place (Bottomley, 1993). This is the basis of the zinc protoporphyrin test (see Chapters 4 and 8). Elevations of erythrocyte protoporphyrin begin to occur at lead levels somewhere between 15 and 18 µg/dL (Piomelli, Seaman, Zullow, Curran, & Davidow, 1982).

ANEMIA

Anemia is a common manifestation of lead poisoning in children. However, it is not a sensitive indicator of lead toxicity and may be absent despite elevated blood lead concentrations. A variety of mechanisms are responsible for the anemia observed in children with lead poisoning. Impaired heme biosynthesis, as described above, is the predominant cause of anemia. Lead also interferes with the synthesis of α- and β-globin chains, which may contribute to anemia (Beutler, 1990). Hemolysis plays a minor role in lead-induced anemia. It results from lead-induced damage to red cell membranes and interference with the cation ATPase pump (Beutler, 1990; Lubran, 1980).

Anemia secondary to iron deficiency is common in children with lead poisoning and is associated with poor nutrition as well as a lead-induced decrease in iron absorption from the gut (Piomelli et al., 1982). Lead may also have an adverse effect on copper metabolism, leading to a sideroblastic anemia that is characteristic of copper deficiency (Klauder & Petering, 1977; Miller et al., 1990).

The anemia of lead poisoning can be normocytic and normochromic but most often is microcytic, hypochromic, and associated with low serum iron levels. However, unlike iron deficiency anemia, lead poisoning anemia is sideroblastic in nature because abnormal accumulations of nonheme iron are located in the mitochondria of red cell precursors (Beutler, 1990; Klauder & Petering, 1977).

Basophilic stippling is another characteristic finding in the erythrocytes of children with lead poisoning. Basophilic stippling represents the accumulation of abnormally aggregated ribosomes that results from impaired RNA degradation. Lead inhibits the activity of 5'-nucleotidase, an enzyme responsible for RNA depolymerization. Although basophilic granules are occasionally seen in patients with lead poisoning, they are not pathognomonic of lead poisoning and the degree of basophilic stippling does not correlate with the severity of the lead burden (Bottomley, 1993).

LEAD AND THE NERVOUS SYSTEM

Central Nervous System Involvement

Among the most controversial and clinically important aspects of plumbism are the effects of lead on the central nervous system (CNS). Children appear to be significantly more susceptible than adults to lead-induced CNS dysfunction. Lower intelligence scores (IQ), learning disabilities, hyperactivity, aggressive and antisocial behavior, attention deficit disorders, autism, hearing and speech impediments, and seizures have all been attributed to elevated lead burdens (see Chapter 6).

It is postulated that lead concentrations at any level may be capable of inducing changes in CNS function (Otto & Reiter, 1984). Altered electrical activity of the brain, as measured by slow-wave cortical potentials, has been observed in children with lead concentrations as low as 15 µg/dL (Otto et al., 1982). The slow wave may be an index of conditioning or learning in children (Otto et al., 1981). These alterations may persist despite subsequent decreases in mean blood lead levels (Otto et al., 1982).

The cerebellum matures more slowly than other parts of the brain and appears to be particularly sensitive to the toxic effects of lead (Winder, Garten, & Lewis, 1983). Evidence of cerebellar edema has been shown on magnetic resonance imaging (MRI) in a 2½-year-old child with lead poisoning (serum lead level 95 µg/dL) who presented with vomiting, abdominal pain, and opisthotonos (Perelman, Hertz-Pannier, Hassan, & Bourrillon, 1993).

Multiple mechanisms of lead neurotoxicity have been proposed (Figure 2). These include effects of lead on the blood–brain barrier, synaptogenesis, heme synthesis, neurotransmitter release, and neuronal activity.

The Blood–Brain Barrier   Lead does not appear to affect the function or the microvasculature of the mature blood–brain barrier in adult rats (Hertz, Bowling, Grandjean, & Westergaard, 1981). However, in immature animals, lead accumulates in CNS mitochondria, capillary

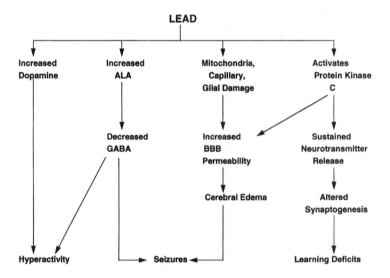

Figure 2.   Effects of lead on the central nervous system. ALA, δ-aminolevulinic acid; GABA, γ-aminobutyric acid; BBB, blood–brain barrier.

endothelial cells, and glia (Silbergeld, 1983). Because of the apparent sensitivity of the neonatal blood–brain barrier to lead, it is postulated that immature astrocytes are incapable of removing endothelial lead, resulting in increased lead uptake, mitochondrial damage, and endothelial necrosis (Goldstein, 1990; Verity, 1990). The resultant changes in microvascular permeability lead to cerebral and cerebellar edema. These effects are associated with the acute encephalopathy observed in patients with high lead levels (usually >70 µg/dL).

Lead may also induce blood–brain barrier damage by activating protein kinases, which are enzymes that are normally stimulated by calcium. Protein kinase C is responsible for transferring a phosphate group from ATP to proteins that regulate membrane channels. The act of phosphorylation changes the configuration of these channels and may consequently affect the permeability of the blood–brain barrier (Goldstein, 1990; Goyer, 1993).

Synaptogenesis   Lead may alter synapse formation and organization. The majority of cerebral neurons develop and migrate to their adult locations during the second trimester of gestation. However, neuronal connections at birth are sparse and relatively inactive, as evidenced by a low cerebral metabolic rate measured by positron emission tomography (Goldstein, 1990). Synaptic density and complexity increase significantly during the first 2 years of life, when lead acquisition is at its peak. By age 3, synaptic density exceeds that of adults, and subsequently a pruning of dendritic arborization takes place with a removal of synapses. The determination of which dendrites and synapses are removed and which remain may be influenced by the amount and complexity of neuronal activity. Protein kinase C is a regulatory enzyme known to affect neuronal activity.

As mentioned earlier, lead at very low concentrations can replace calcium in the activation of protein kinase C. In nerve terminals, activated protein kinase C phosphorylates proteins that promote neurotransmitter release. Prolonged activation of protein kinase C from chronic lead exposure can cause sustained neurotransmitter release. The consequential loss of normal controlled neuronal activity may affect synaptic development (Goldstein, 1990). Lead exposure in the developing rat brain results in a decrease in the number of synapses and neurotransmitter receptors (Regan, 1992). It is conceivable that the associated decreased density of synapses or the inefficient manner in which they develop may be related to learning deficits and diminished cognitive function previously reported.

Lead and Neurotransmitters   As described earlier in the section on heme synthesis, patients with lead poisoning have an increased production of ALA. ALA inhibits the release of the CNS inhibitory neurotransmitter γ-aminobutyric acid (GABA). ALA may also compete with GABA at synaptic membranes (Hermes-Lima et al., 1991; Silbergeld, 1982). The absence of the inhibitory effects of GABA may at least partially explain the increased seizure sensitivity and perhaps the hyperactivity observed in patients with severe lead intoxication (Silbergeld, Miller, Kennedy, & Eng, 1979). Although the breakdown of the blood–brain barrier may contribute to a lowered seizure threshold, the convulsant properties of lead have also been observed in animals without evidence of blood–brain barrier disruption (Silbergeld et al., 1979).

Lead exposure also influences catecholamine and acetylcholine release (Silbergeld et al., 1979). In lead poisoning, calcium-dependent acetylcholine release is decreased (Silbergeld & Adler, 1978), whereas dopamine synthesis is reduced in some areas of the brain and increased in others (Govoni, Memo, Spano, & Trabucchi, 1979). Those areas of increased dopamine release may offer another explanation for the hyperactive behavior observed in many patients with lead poisoning. Elevated urinary concentrations of the dopamine metabolite homovanillic acid (HVA) have been associated with lead levels of 40 µg/100 mL and higher (Beritic, 1981).

Peripheral Nervous System Involvement

Children primarily manifest evidence of CNS dysfunction, whereas the presentation of lead poisoning in adults mainly involves peripheral neuropathy. Peripheral nervous system abnormalities are rare in children. If they occur, they usually present 2–3 months after CNS manifestations (DeMichele, 1984; McCabe, 1979; Seppalainen, 1982). However, there have been documented instances of lead neuropathy in children without coexistent encephalopathy (Beritic, 1981). Symptoms of lead-induced peripheral neuropathy in children include generalized weakness, diaphragmatic paralysis, footdrop, and wrist drop (Wong, Ng, & Yeung, 1991). Furthermore, evidence of subclinical neuropathy, manifested by slowed peroneal motor nerve conduction velocities, has been demonstrated in children with lead levels of 40 mg/100 g or greater (Feldman, Hayes, Younes, & Aldrich, 1977). Sensation appears to be unaffected (Beritic, 1981).

Lead neuropathy may result from damage to a variety of structures including blood vessels, Schwann cells, stromal cells, and nerve cells. Another proposed mechanism involves the effect of lead on demyelination (Figure 3). As the reader will recall, Schwann cells and stromal cells are responsible for myelin formation. Lead may disturb calcium transport resulting in Schwann cell swelling and damage (Whetsell, Sassa, & Kappas, 1984). Lead also affects mitochondrial oxidative phosphorylation; consequently, some of the observed Schwann cell

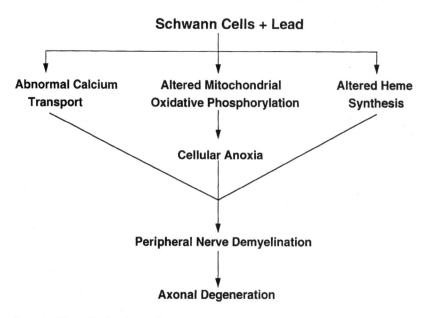

Figure 3. Effects of lead on the peripheral nervous system.

changes may represent cellular anoxia (Brashear, Kopp, & Krigman, 1978). Finally, heme production occurs within these cells and appears to be essential for the metabolic processes involved in myelin development. Lead-induced impairment of heme formation results in segmental degeneration of myelin sheaths in peripheral neurons in mice (Whetsell et al., 1984). Axonal damage appears to be secondary to impaired myelin formation and occurs only if demyelination is severe (Beritic, 1981).

Another theory is that of the "dying back" mechanism of motor neuron disease. Metabolic processes in neurons are dependent on successful transport of protoplasm, proteins, and other nutrients from the perikaryon (the axon body) outwardly to the tips of the axons. It is hypothesized that lead may interfere with this process by affecting the synthesis or the transport of these nutrients (Beritic, 1981).

Autonomic Nervous System Involvement

Lead affects parasympathetic activity by decreasing acetylcholine release at preganglionic nerve endings and at the neuromuscular junction (Janin, Couinaud, Stone, & Wise, 1985; Keate, DiPietrantonio, & Randleman, 1983; Murata, Araki, Yokoyama, Uchida, & Fujimura, 1993). The alterations in parasympathetic activity are manifested primarily by changes in smooth muscle tone. In addition, the gastrointestinal symptoms observed in lead-poisoned patients are thought to be related to abnormalities within the autonomic nervous system (see next section).

Lead-calcium competition may be responsible for the anticholinergic effects of lead. Lead may competitively inhibit calcium entry into presynaptic nerve terminals (Janin et al., 1985). This is supported by the clinical observation that calcium has a beneficial effect on lead colic (Beritic, 1981).

GASTROINTESTINAL SYMPTOMS OF LEAD POISONING

Lead colic is a common presenting manifestation of lead poisoning. It is usually associated with blood lead levels greater than 60 µg/dL (Ellenhorn & Barceloux, 1988). The abdominal symptoms observed in lead-poisoned patients can be paroxysmal but are frequently constant; hence the term *lead colic* is a misnomer. The pain may be localized or diffuse, and vomiting may or may not be present. Furthermore, vomiting can be a manifestation of intra-abdominal processes or intracranial abnormalities such as cerebral edema. The physical examination may reveal localized or diffuse abdominal tenderness, or, by contrast, the pain may diminish with palpation (Janin et al., 1985). Abdominal guarding or rigidity may be present in a minority of patients; however, gross distention of the abdomen is exceedingly uncharacteristic. The abdominal symptoms and physical findings observed in children with lead poisoning are thought to result from the effects of lead on the autonomic nervous system as described above.

Constipation is also common in children with lead poisoning. One proposed mechanism for this finding results from the observation that lead interferes with sodium-potassium-ATPase activity in the small intestine. Resultant alterations in sodium transport may promote water flux abnormalities and thus result in constipation (Janin et al., 1985). Diarrhea can also occur, but is less frequent.

Lead-induced abdominal pain has been confused with acute intestinal obstruction, acute appendicitis, and acute cholecystitis. Other, less common misdiagnoses include anorexia nervosa, pyloric stenosis, mesenteric thrombosis, and acute porphyria (Janin et al., 1985). In fact, the major symptoms of hereditary impairments of heme biosynthesis and porphyrin accumulation (e.g., abdominal pain, constipation, neuropathy) closely resemble those of lead poisoning.

Abdominal radiographs of patients with lead intoxication and abdominal pain may be normal or may show dilated loops with or without air fluid levels. Upper gastrointestinal radiologic examinations performed on patients with lead poisoning and vomiting have shown gastric contractions, pyloric spasm, and gastric retention. Atony, dilated small-intestinal loops, and delays in transit time have all been demonstrated in small bowel studies. Barium enema studies have found in some patients functional megacolon that was either localized or diffuse (Janin et al., 1985). Symptoms and radiographic abnormalities resolve with treatment of the lead poisoning.

LEAD IN BONE

Bone as a Storage Site for Lead

Bone is the major repository for lead in the body (Markowitz & Weinberger, 1990). The amount of lead stored in bone increases with age. In children, skeletal bone carries approximately 70% of the total body lead burden (Mushak, 1993). In the adult, over 95% of the lead stored in the body is located in bone (Weeden, 1992). Bone lead accumulation begins during fetal development and continues up to about age 60 years (Pounds, Long, & Rosen, 1991). The rates of accumulation are dependent on the degree of lead exposure and the skeletal site (Rabinowitz, 1991).

The indices most commonly used to determine the efficacy of chelating agents to rid the body of lead—the serum lead and erythrocyte protoporphyrin levels—do not reflect the total amount of lead stored in bone. X-ray fluorescence is a noninvasive technique that can identify lead sequestered in bone (Weeden, 1992). Fluorescence of K-shell electrons can provide a measurement of whole-bone lead. K-fluorescent X-rays are capable of measuring lead as deep as 2 cm, a depth similar to that obtained in biopsy specimens. L-fluorescent X-rays penetrate only the outer 0.5 mm of periosteal bone and consequently allow for the measurement of lead located on the surface of bone.

Bone as a Source of Lead Exposure

Lead that was accumulated in bone was originally thought to be permanently removed from the circulation. It is now known, however, that lead stored in bone can potentially provide a continuous source of lead exposure to other organs. Although chelation therapy with ethylenediaminetetraacetic acid (EDTA) is capable of removing significant amounts of lead from bone, some lead is stored in a manner that makes it unavailable for removal by this method. Lead that penetrates the crystalline surface of bone remains buried until osteoclast turnover allows for bone remodeling and lead mobilization (Rabinowitz, 1991).

The rate of bone turnover also depends on the skeletal site and the age of the patient. For example, the tibia, fibula, femur, and skull turn over at a rate of about 2% per year (Rabinowitz, 1991). The spine turns over at a rate approximating 8% per year. As expected, young children have a higher turnover rate than adults: 85% per year during the first year of life, 7% per year in the 20s, and 2% per year in the 30s. After age 60, rates increase again to over 4% per year.

Lead is incorporated into and released from bone in a manner that parallels calcium metabolism. Factors that influence the storage and release of calcium are likely to affect the storage and release of bone lead. Thus, changes in acid–base equilibrium will alter rates of bone lead mobilization (Finkel et al., 1983). As expected, conditions that promote bone remodeling and osteoporosis also stimulate lead release from bone. In fact, large increases in blood lead, erythrocyte protoporphyrin, and ionized calcium concentrations have been observed in children following bone fractures and inactivity during hospitalization (Markowitz & Weinberger, 1990).

The release of lead from bone repositories may have important consequences. Mobilization of maternal bone lead may occur during the later stages of pregnancy and can be a significant source of lead to the fetus (Markowitz & Weinberger, 1990; Silbergeld et al., 1993). The kinetics of lead exchange between blood, bone, and soft tissue are variable. Therefore, a single, prenatal serum lead level may not be an adequate screen for potential fetal lead exposure (Mushak, 1993). As discussed previously, the effects of chronic lead exposure on the nervous system can be significant. The effects of lead on the kidney as discussed below, and its potential effect on other organs, can frequently be attributed to chronic exposure to lead released from storage sites in bone.

Effects of Lead on Bone

In addition to being deposited in bones, lead interferes with bone formation, bone maturation, and bone resorption. Consequently, lead poisoning can potentially alter bone structure and bone size. As observed in other organ systems, the developing skeleton is more sensitive to lead toxicity than the adult skeleton. Lead readily crosses the placenta and can produce congenital skeletal anomalies. Fetal lead exposure in rats, mice, and hamsters has been associated with fusion of two or more vertebrae in the anterior part of the axial skeleton (Pounds et al., 1991). Similarly, studies examining human congenital lead poisoning have described delayed skeletal and deciduous teeth development at birth (Pounds et al., 1991). Radiographs of these children 7 months after chelation therapy revealed normal maturation but delayed tooth eruption until 15 months of age.

Lead appears to affect postnatal bone development as well. High concentrations of lead have caused a condition similar to rickets in children (Silbergeld et al., 1993). Studies reviewing lower-level lead exposure have observed an inverse relationship between blood lead concentrations and height and chest circumference in children younger than 7 years of age (Pounds et al., 1991; Silbergeld et al., 1993).

Lead affects bone development directly by altering bone cell function and indirectly by altering hormonal mediators of bone production. The combination of these effects results in abnormal bone formation and resorption.

Lead and Bone Cell Activity Lead alters bone formation by incorporating into and inhibiting the formation of the mineral matrix of bone. Lead also interferes with bone resorption, presumably by damaging osteoclasts. Histologically, lead-containing inclusion bodies are found in the cytoplasm and nuclei of osteoclasts but are not found in osteoblasts or osteocytes. These inclusion bodies have also been identified in the kidney and the liver and are thought to be pathognomonic for lead poisoning (Pounds et al., 1991).

Lead and Hormonal Regulation of Bone Cell Activity Patients with lead poisoning have alterations in a number of the hormones responsible for regulating bone cell activity. Lead may also alter the bone cell's ability to respond to hormonal regulation. The active form of vitamin D, 1,25-dihydroxy vitamin D_3, plays an important role in bone growth, bone mineralization, cell differentiation, cell maturation, and immunoregulation. Parathyroid hormone is an important stimulator of bone resorption. Decreased circulating levels of 1,25-dihydroxy vitamin D_3 and increased blood levels of parathyroid hormone have been described in children with lead levels of 15–20 µg/dL (Kaminsky et al., 1993; Mahaffey et al., 1982; Pounds et al., 1991).

LEAD AND RENAL DYSFUNCTION/HYPERTENSION

Acute severe lead intoxication can cause disorders in proximal tubular transport characteristic of Fanconi's syndrome. Abnormalities include excessive urinary losses of amino acids, glucose, phosphate, potassium, bicarbonate, and low molecular weight proteins. One or more of these findings may be absent if the expression of this syndrome is incomplete. Histologically, round acidophilic intranuclear inclusion bodies are found in the proximal tubule and loops of Henle (Ellenhorn & Barceloux, 1988). Renal dysfunction during childhood lead poisoning is usually reversible (Ellenhorn & Barceloux, 1988).

Although lead poisoning in chronically exposed adults has been linked to hypertension and chronic lead nephropathy, such associations in children remain controversial. Inglis, Henderson, and Emmerson (1978) described untreated children with lead poisoning in

Queensland, Australia, who developed hypertension and chronic renal insufficiency in adulthood. They postulated that the sequence of events leading to renal failure involved glomerular destruction during childhood lead poisoning followed by resolution of the destruction later in childhood and adolescence and by the onset of hypertension and chronic uremia in late adolescence or early adulthood. This sequence was not complete in milder cases (Inglis et al., 1978).

Jhaveri et al. (1979) reported elevated systolic blood pressures in infants and children with blood lead concentrations greater than 40 µg/dL. In this study, the median systolic blood pressure was 94 mm Hg in patients with blood lead levels greater than 40 µg/dL and 74 mm Hg in those with blood lead levels of 40 µg/dL and less. However, most investigators have found no evidence of impairment of renal function or hypertension in children following treatment for lead poisoning (Friedlander, 1981; Moel & Sachs, 1992; Moel, Sachs, Cohn, & Drayton, 1985; Rogan, Hogan, & Chi, 1978). Moel and coworkers postulate that the absence of findings may reflect an inadequate amount of time allowed for evidence of renal nephropathy to develop. As indicated above, lead accumulations in bone remain metabolically active and can exert multisystem effects for years. In the Queensland patients, the lead content of bone was higher in those with renal disease than in those without renal disease (Inglis et al., 1978). It has been theorized that renal exposure to chronically high levels of lead released from significant bone stores is necessary for chronic renal failure to develop. Hu (1991) found support for this theory and described an increased occurrence of hypertension and elevated creatinine clearance in survivors of childhood lead poisoning 50 years after exposure to lead.

AUDITORY AND LANGUAGE DYSFUNCTION

Lead exposure has also been shown to impair auditory function. Increased hearing thresholds have been observed in children with blood lead levels as low as 10 µg/dL (Otto & Fox, 1993; Schwartz & Otto, 1991). Cranial nerve VIII appears to be the target involved in lead-induced hearing abnormalities (Otto & Fox, 1993). Brain stem auditory evoked potentials (BAEP) are often used to evaluate cochlear nerve dysfunction and nonspecific demyelinating diseases (Otto & Fox, 1993). Increased latencies in BAEP have been observed in lead-exposed children (Otto & Fox, 1993). High-dose lead exposure in the adult guinea pig has caused 1) histologic evidence of cochlear nerve damage, including segmental demyelination and axonal degeneration, and 2) a decrease in the maximum amplitude of the nerve action potential (Otto & Fox, 1993).

Abnormal language-related behaviors have also been observed in lead-exposed children (Dietrich, Succop, Berger, & Keith, 1992; Needleman et al., 1979; White, Diamond, Proctor, Morey, & Hu, 1993). Blood lead levels above 11.5 µg/dL have been associated with delayed language development (Schwartz & Otto, 1987). These abnormalities may result from hearing impairments but can also occur despite normal hearing sensitivity. Disorders in auditory and language processing may account for this finding because patients with auditory processing abnormalities have difficulty perceiving language when the signal is less than optimal, despite normal hearing sensitivity and normal intelligence (Dietrich et al., 1992). Such suboptimal situations are frequently encountered in noisy classrooms. Both impaired auditory processing and increased hearing thresholds may contribute to childhood learning disorders and delays in attainment of developmental milestones.

VISUAL DYSFUNCTION

A myriad of visual symptoms have been attributed to lead poisoning, including amblyopia, blindness, scotomatas, eye muscle paralysis, ptosis, cataracts, mydriasis, and optic neuritis or atrophy (Otto & Fox, 1993). Impaired spatial and temporal resolution has also been described in children with lead poisoning. These impairments include a decreased ability to discriminate size and to detect the direction and speed of movements (Fox, Wright, & Costa, 1982). Studies of newborn rats exposed to lead have shown decreased visual acuity (Fox et al., 1982).

Newborn rats fed subclinical doses of lead (defined in this study as doses that do not induce overt neurologic disturbances) have displayed evidence of focal retinal necrosis without damage to retinal vessels (Santos-Anderson, Tso, Valdes, & Annau, 1984). Neonatal exposure to blood lead concentrations of 59 µg/dL has resulted specifically in rod cell degeneration without affecting cone cells in rats (Fox & Katz, 1991). Rod cell dysfunction in rats has been demonstrated at blood lead levels less than 20 µg/dL (Otto & Fox, 1993), although to date rod cell function in lead-exposed children has not been examined.

Neonatal lead exposure also alters visual cholinergic muscarinic receptor binding and density in rats. These effects are specific to the visual cortex and spare the retinal structures (Costa & Fox, 1983; Fox et al., 1982).

CARDIAC EFFECTS OF LEAD

Most studies involving lead cardiotoxicity focus on the rat or mouse model. However, there have been clinical reports of sudden death in patients who received lead-contaminated intravenous solutions (Williams, Hejtmancik, & Abreu, 1983). Although the reports are few, the potential consequences of acutely high or chronically low cardiac lead exposure may be critical.

Reported cardiac effects in rats fed or perfused with lead include negative inotropism, cardiomyopathy, conduction defects (specifically PR prolongation and heart block), and increased sensitivity to the arrhythmogenic effect of norepinephrine. The negative inotropism observed is thought to result from a lead-induced abnormality in calcium transport. Cardiomyopathy with myocardial ultrastructural changes has been observed in mice at lead levels less than 40 µg/dL. Conduction defects are secondary to the effects of lead on the His-Purkinje system.

An adult onset increased sensitivity to the arrhythmogenic action of norepinephrine was demonstrated when newborn rats were fed lead acetate in drinking water at birth. These effects were pronounced at 3 months of age, after a lead-free period when the heart lead concentrations had dropped to control levels. Cutting of the vagus nerve abolishes this phenomenon; consequently, increased parasympathetic activity is thought to play a role. As described above, lead decreases GABA release. Under normal circumstances, GABA decreases vagal activity. A lead-induced decrease in GABA is therefore postulated to account for the increase in parasympathetic activity and the observed cardiosensitivity to norepinephrine in lead-exposed animals.

ORAL MANIFESTATIONS OF LEAD POISONING

Oral manifestations of chronic lead poisoning include stomatitis, sialorrhea with swelling of the salivary glands, metallic taste, dysphagia, a heavy coating on the tongue, and tongue tremors (Lockhart, 1981). Another interesting finding in 20%–85% of all patients with lead poisoning is a gingival pigmentation known as a "lead line" or "Burtonian line." This line is characterized by a 1- to 3-mm bluish black or slate gray line at the gingival margin. Similar lines can also be seen in patients with bismuth and mercury poisoning. The differential diagnosis includes gingivitis, normal pigmentation, and discoloration due to amalgam tattoo.

Lead lines occur in areas of localized trauma or irritation and represent subendothelial depositions of lead sulfide. Lead compounds leak through inflamed areas of increased permeability and react with hydrogen sulfide (released from anaerobic organisms around teeth) to form lead sulfide. Lead lines have become less common through the years as dental hygiene has improved. They do not appear in patients with adequate oral hygiene, in infants, and in edentulous patients.

CONCLUSIONS

The effects of high-level lead exposure can be devastating, with potential influences on multiple organ systems. The effects of low-level lead exposure may also produce organ system abnormalities, although the manifestations may be subtle or subclinical. It is difficult, however, to assess the potential consequences of lost IQ points, decreased hearing, and impaired visual acuity. The long-term sequelae of childhood low-level lead exposure, as they pertain to adult social skills and job acquisition or performance, have not been adequately studied and remain unknown. Further investigation is required before subclinical effects of subtoxic blood lead levels can be dismissed as inconsequential.

REFERENCES

Barltrop, D., & Meek, F. (1979). Effect of particle size on lead absorption from the gut. *Archives of Environmental Health, 34,* 280–285.

Beck, W. (Ed.). (1981). *Hematology* (3rd ed.). Cambridge, MA: MIT Press.

Beritic, T. (1981). Lead neuropathy. *Critical Review in Toxicology, 12,* 149–213.

Beutler, E. (1990). Hemolytic anemia due to chemical and physical agents. In W. Williams, E. Beutler, A. Erslev, & M. Lichtman (Eds.), *Hematology* (pp. 660–662). New York: McGraw-Hill.

Biddle, G. (1982). Toxicology of lead: Primer for analytical chemists. *Association of Official Analytical Chemistry, 65,* 947–952.

Bottomley, S. (1993). Sideroblastic anemias. In G. Lee, T. Bithell, J. Foerster, J. Athens, & J. Lukens (Eds.), *Wintrobe's clinical hematology* (pp. 863–865). Philadelphia: Lea and Febiger.

Brashear, C., Kopp, V., & Krigman, M. (1978). Effect of lead on the developing peripheral nervous system. *Journal of Neuropathology and Experimental Neurology, 37,* 414–425.

Chisolm, J., Angle, C., Bornschein, R., Graziano, J., Keck, J., Mortensen, M., & Needleman, H. (1991). *A new look at lead toxicity: Conference on childhood lead toxicity* [pamphlet]. Comtack Corporation.

Costa, L., & Fox, D. (1983). A selective decrease of cholinergic muscarinic receptors in the visual cortex of adult rats following developmental lead exposure. *Brain Research, 276,* 259–266.

DeMichele, S. (1984). Nutrition of lead. *Comparative Biochemistry and Physiology, 78A,* 401–408.

Dietrich, K., Succop, P., Berger, O., & Keith, R. (1992). Lead exposure and the central auditory processing abilities and cognitive development of urban children: The Cincinnati lead study cohort at age 5 years. *Neurotoxicology and Teratology, 14,* 51–56.

Ellenhorn, M., & Barceloux, D. (Eds.). (1988). *Medical toxicology* (1st ed.). New York: Elsevier.

Feldman, R., Hayes, M., Younes, R., & Aldrich, F. (1977). Lead neuropathy in adults and children. *Archives of Neurology, 34,* 481–488.

Finkel, A., Hamilton, A., & Hardy, H. (1983). Lead. In A. Finkel (Ed.), *Hamilton and Hardy's industrial toxicology* (4th ed., pp. 62–87). Boston: John Wright & Sons Ltd.

Fox, D., & Katz, L. (1991). Low level developmental lead exposure decreases the sensitivity, amplitude and temporal resolution of rods. *Neurotoxicology, 12,* 641–654.

Fox, D., Wright, A., & Costa, L. (1982). Visual acuity deficits following neonatal lead exposure: Cholinergic interactions. *Neurobehavioral Toxicology and Teratology, 4,* 689–693.

Friedlander, M. (1981). Blood pressure and creatinine clearance in lead-exposed children: The effect of treatment. *Archives of Environmental Health, 36,* 310–315.

Goering, P. (1993). Lead-protein interactions as a basis for lead toxicity. *Neurotoxicology, 14,* 45–60.

Goldstein, G. (1990). Lead poisoning and brain cell function. *Environmental Health Perspectives, 89,* 91–94.

Govoni, S., Memo, M., Spano, P., & Trabucchi, M. (1979). Chronic lead treatment differentially affects dopamine synthesis in various rat brain areas. *Toxicology, 12,* 343–349.

Goyer, R. (1993). Lead toxicity: Current concerns. *Environmental Health Perspectives, 100,* 177–187.

Graef, J. (1992). Lead poisoning. *Clinical Toxicology Review, 14,* 1–6.

Hermes-Lima, M., Pereira, B., & Bechara, J. (1991). Are free radicals involved in lead poisoning? *Xenobiotica, 21,* 1085–1090.

Hertz, M., Bowling, T., Grandjean, P., & Westergaard, E. (1981). Lead poisoning and the blood–brain barrier. *Acta Neurologica Scandinavia, 63,* 286–296.

Hu, H. (1991). A 50 year follow-up of childhood plumbism. *American Journal of the Diseases of Children, 145,* 681–687.

Inglis, J., Henderson, D., & Emmerson, B. (1978). The pathology and pathogenesis of chronic lead nephropathy occurring in Queensland. *Journal of Pathology, 124,* 65–76.

Janin, Y., Couinaud, C., Stone, A., & Wise, L. (1985). The "lead-induced colic" syndrome in lead intoxication. *Surgical Annals, 17,* 287–307.

Jhaveri, R., Lavorgna, L., Dube, S., Glass, L., Khan, F., & Evans, H. (1979). Relationship of blood pressure to blood lead concentrations in small children. *Pediatrics, 63,* 674–676.

Kaminsky, P., Klein, M., & Duc, M. (1993). Physiopathologie de l'intoxication par le plomb inorganique. *La Revue de Medecine Interne, 14,* 163–170.

Keate, R., DiPietrantonio, P., & Randleman, M. (1983). Occupational lead exposure. *Annals of Emergency Medicine, 12,* 786–788.

Klauder, D., & Petering, H. (1977). Anemia of lead intoxication: A role for copper. *Journal of Nutrition, 107,* 1779–1785.

Lockhart, P.B. (1981). Gingival pigmentation as the sole presenting sign of chronic lead poisoning in a mentally retarded adult. *Oral Surgery, 52,* 143–149.

Lubran, M. (1980). Lead toxicity and heme biosynthesis. *Annals of Clinical and Laboratory Science, 10,* 402–413.

Mahaffey, K., Rosen, J., Chesney, R., Peeler, J., Smith, C., & DeLuca, H. (1982). Association between age, blood lead concentration, and serum 1,25-dihydroxycholecalciferol levels in children. *American Journal of Clinical Nutrition, 35,* 1327–1331.

Markowitz, M., & Weinberger, H. (1990). Immobilization-related lead toxicity in previously lead-poisoned children. *Pediatrics, 86,* 455–456.

McCabe, E. (1979). Age and sensitivity to lead toxicity: A review. *Environmental Health Perspectives, 29,* 29–33.

McColl, K., & Goldberg, A. (1980). Abnormal porphyrin metabolism in diseases other than porphyria. *Clinics in Haematology, 9*, 427–444.

Meredith, P., Moore, M., Campbell, B., Thompson, G., & Goldberg, A. (1978). Delta-aminolaevulinic acid metabolism in normal and lead-exposed humans. *Toxicology, 9*, 1–9.

Miller, G., Massaro, T., & Massaro, E. (1990). Interactions between lead and essential elements: A review. *Neurotoxicology, 11*, 99–120.

Moel, D., & Sachs, H. (1992). Renal function 17 to 23 years after chelation therapy for childhood plumbism. *Kidney International, 42*, 1226–1231.

Moel, D., Sachs, H., Cohn, R., & Drayton, M. (1985). Renal function 9–17 years after childhood lead poisoning. *Journal of Pediatrics, 106*, 729–733.

Morrow, P., Beiter, H., Amato, F., & Gibb, F. (1980). Pulmonary retention of lead: An experimental study in man. *Environmental Research, 21*, 373–384.

Murata, K., Araki, S., Yokoyama, K., Uchida, E., & Fujimura, Y. (1993). Assessment of central, peripheral, autonomic nervous system functions in lead workers: Neuroelectrophysiological studies. *Environmental Research, 61*, 323–336.

Mushak, P. (1993). New directions in the toxicokinetics of human lead exposure. *Neurotoxicology, 14*, 29–42.

Needleman, R., Gunnoe, C., Leviton, A., Reed, R., Peresie, H., Maher, C., & Barrett, P. (1979). Deficits in psychologic and classroom performance of children with elevated dentine lead levels. *New England Journal of Medicine, 300*, 689–695.

Otto, D., Benignus, V., Muller, K., & Barton, C. (1981). Effects of age and body lead burden on CNS function in young children. I. Slow cortical potentials. *Electroencephalography and Clinical Neurophysiology, 52*, 229–239.

Otto, D., Benignus, V., Muller, K., Seiple, K., Prah, J., & Schroeder, S. (1982). Effects of low to moderate lead exposure on slow cortical potentials in young children: Two year follow-up study. *Neurobehavioral Toxicology and Teratology, 4*, 733–737.

Otto, D., & Fox, D. (1993). Auditory and visual dysfunction following lead exposure. *Neurotoxicology, 14*, 191–208.

Otto, D., & Reiter, L. (1984). Developmental changes in slow cortical potentials of young children with elevated body lead burdens. *Annals of the New York Academy of Sciences, 425*, 377–383.

Perelman, S., Hertz-Pannier, L., Hassan, M., & Bourrillon, A. (1993). Lead encephalopathy mimicking a cerebellar tumor. *Acta Paediatrics, 82*, 423–425.

Piomelli, S., Seaman, C., Zullow, D., Curran, A., & Davidow, B. (1982). Threshold for lead damage to heme synthesis in urban children. *Proceedings of the National Academy of Science, 79*, 3335–3339.

Pounds, J., Long, G., & Rosen, J. (1991). Cellular and molecular toxicity of lead in bone. *Environmental Health Perspectives, 91*, 17–32.

Rabinowitz, M. (1991). Toxicokinetics of bone lead. *Environmental Health Perspectives, 91*, 33–37.

Regan, C. (1992). Neural cell adhesion molecules, neuronal development and lead toxicity. *Neurotoxicology, 14*, 69–74.

Regan, H. (1983). The bioavailability of iron, lead and cadmium via gastrointestinal absorption. *Science of the Total Environment, 28*, 317–326.

Rogan, W., Hogan, M., & Chi, P. (1978). Blood pressure and lead levels in children. *Journal of Environmental Pathology and Toxicology, 2*, 517–519.

Rosenstock, L., & Cullen, M. (1986). Metals. In J. Dyson (Ed.), *Clinical occupational medicine* (pp. 205–207). Philadelphia: W.B. Saunders.

Santos-Anderson, R., Tso, M., Valdes, J., & Annau, Z. (1984). Chronic lead administration in neonatal rats: Electron microscopy of the retina. *Journal of Neuropathology and Experimental Neurology, 43,* 175–187.

Schwartz, J., & Otto, D. (1987). Blood lead, hearing thresholds, and neurobehavioral development in children and youth. *Archives of Environmental Health, 42,* 153–160.

Schwartz, J., & Otto, D. (1991). Lead and minor hearing impairment. *Archives of Environmental Health, 46,* 300–305.

Seppalainen, A. (1982). Lead poisoning: Neurophysiological aspects. *Acta Neurologica Scandinavia, 66,* 177–184.

Silbergeld, E. (1982). Effects of altered porphyrin synthesis in brain neurochemistry. *Neurobehavioral Toxicology and Teratology, 4,* 635–642.

Silbergeld, E. (1983). Localization of metals: Issues of importance to neurotoxicology of lead. *Neurotoxicology, 4,* 193–200.

Silbergeld, E., & Adler, H. (1978). Subcellular mechanisms of lead neurotoxicity. *Brain Research, 148,* 451–467.

Silbergeld, E., Miller, L., Kennedy, S., & Eng, N. (1979). Lead, GABA, and seizures: Effects of subencephalopathic lead exposures on seizure sensitivity and GABAergic function. *Environmental Research, 19,* 371–382.

Silbergeld, E., Sauk, J., Somerman, M., Todd, A., McNeill, F., Fowler, B., Fontaine, A., & Van Buren, J. (1993). Lead in bone: Storage site, exposure source, and target organ. *Neurotoxicology, 14,* 225–236.

Verity, M. (1990). Comparative observations on inorganic and organic lead neurotoxicity. *Environmental Health Perspectives, 89,* 43–48.

Weeden, R. (1992). Removing lead from bone: Clinical implications of bone lead stores. *Neurotoxicology, 13,* 843–852.

Whetsell, W., Sassa, S., & Kappas, A. (1984). Porphyrin-heme biosynthesis in organotypic cultures of mouse dorsal root ganglia. Effects of heme and lead on porphyrin synthesis and peripheral myelin. *Journal of Clinical Investigation, 74,* 600–607.

White, R., Diamond, R., Proctor, S., Morey, C., & Hu, H. (1993). Residual cognitive deficits 50 years after lead poisoning during childhood. *British Journal of Industrial Medicine, 50,* 613–622.

Williams, B., Hejtmancik, M., & Abreu, M. (1983). Cardiac effects of lead. *Federation Proceedings, 42,* 2989–2993.

Winder, C., Garten, L., & Lewis, P. (1983). The morphological effects of lead on the developing central nervous system. *Neuropathology and Applied Neurobiology, 9,* 87–108.

Wong, V., Ng, T., & Yeung, C. (1991). Electrophysiologic study in acute lead poisoning. *Pediatric Neurology, 7,* 133–136.

6

LEARNING AND BEHAVIORAL SEQUELAE OF LEAD POISONING

David Bellinger

S ystematic research on the effects of lead on children's behavior and development began in the 1940s (Byers & Lord, 1943) and has continued unabated into the 1990s (Pounds, Cory-Slechta, & Cranmer, 1993). The evolution in the epidemiologic designs employed in these efforts has followed a common pattern. Descriptive studies of case series of clinically lead-poisoned children were followed by case-control, cohort, and prospective studies of children with milder forms of intoxication and, most recently, by quasi-experimental studies of the efficacy of medical or environmental interventions in reducing lead-associated neurobehavioral morbidity (Bellinger & Stiles, 1993).

One of the least controversial statements that can be made about these studies is that their interpretation has been attended by controversy that at times was quite bitter. There are many reasons for this. Within the realm of science, one can point to a number of methodologic challenges in drawing inferences from epidemiologic studies of exposure–outcome relationships. One class of problem involves exposure assessment, in particular the difficulty of assembling accurate and detailed histories of children's lead exposure. It is not possible to measure delivered dose at the critical target tissue for neurotoxicity (brain), resulting in the need to rely on peripheral markers of internal exposure (e.g., blood lead, tooth lead, hair lead). Some biologic exposure markers have such short half-lives that they convey relatively little information about key aspects of the "dosing regimen" that characterizes a child's exposure history and that must be known in order to establish dose-effect or dose-response relationships. Lack of information about these temporal characteristics of exposure increases the difficulty of applying one of the cardinal criteria for evaluating whether an epidemiologic association reflects a causal process (i.e., occurrence of the putative cause, lead exposure, before the putative effect, developmental impairment).

Another class of methodologic problem issues from the fact that all research on lead's effects on children's growth and development is necessarily observational rather than experimental. From a scientific standpoint, it is unfortunate that lead exposure is not randomly distributed among children, but rather tends to co-occur with other exposures, events, and conditions that are risk factors for adverse development. This creates fertile ground for the commission of both Type I errors (i.e., attributing to lead an effect that is more properly attributed to a confounding risk factor such as low social class) and Type II errors (i.e, failing to appreciate lead-associated performance differences within the "statistical noise" contributed by the impact of correlated risk factors on development).

Nevertheless, perhaps in part because of the controversy, important advances have been made in the rigor of the methods used to address these methodologic challenges. As discussed by Bellinger and Dietrich (in press), four advances warrant particular mention. First, exposure history has been characterized more comprehensively. The design of many recent studies incorporated serial prospective assessments of children's blood lead levels at frequent intervals over the first years of life. In addition, substantial effort has been invested in developing methods for sampling body compartments or pools with different exposure averaging times (e.g., tooth, bone, blood plasma) and in developing more comprehensive models of lead biokinetics. Improved quality assurance and quality control procedures for collecting, storing, and analyzing samples have produced more valid and precise blood lead measurements, an issue that becomes increasingly important as the magnitude of the blood lead levels prompting concern decreases (Flegal & Smith, 1992).

A second area of methodologic improvement is outcome assessment. Case-control studies were not designed to identify subtle lead-associated dysfunctions. They sought instead to assess the prevalence of elevated lead burdens among clinic-based samples of children already carrying clinical diagnoses such as "hyperactivity," "learning disability," or "minimal brain dysfunction." Later cross-sectional and prospective studies have generally recruited "normal" children without developmental diagnoses, often using community-based sampling procedures. In most such studies, IQ and educational achievement tests have served as the developmental or cognitive end points. Although useful as bases for formulating public policy, such indices are crude and shed relatively little light on the neuropsychological mechanisms or the brain–behavior relationships underlying lead-associated dysfunction (Bellinger, 1995b; Bernstein, 1994).

More assiduous attempts to measure potential confounders and to adjust for them statistically represents a third area of methodologic improvement (Ruff & Bijur, 1989). Unfortunately, ineluctable constraints imposed by the observational design of these studies limit the extent to which this problem can be eliminated. As a result, animal models, especially those involving primates, assume critical importance in evaluating the likelihood that lead exposure causes cognitive dysfunction (Rice, 1992a). The random assignment of animals to exposure strata reduces the likelihood that any apparent lead effects are confounded by other exposures or events. However, uncertainty about the generalizability of exposure–outcome relationships across species remains a major obstacle.

A fourth type of methodologic advance, closely associated with the third, is the increasing use of sophisticated statistical methods. Whereas many older studies involved straightforward T-test comparisons of the performance of children classified simply as "exposed" or "nonexposed," recent studies have employed multivariate statistical techniques that make greater use of available information (e.g., structural equation modeling, optimal regression, and nonparametric smoothing analysis). Moreover, statistical methods to address issues such as measurement error, confounder misclassification, model specification, and model building have also been introduced.

In the following sections, current data on lead and various functional domains are discussed: intelligence, academic achievement, and "learning disabilities," as well as psychiatric and behavioral disorders. This is followed by a discussion of whether lead-associated cognitive effects resolve, either with the passage of time or as the result of medical or environmental interventions that reduce body lead burden.

INTELLIGENCE

Children's intelligence (operationalized as IQ) is the end point that served as the focus of much of the debate over lead's effects at low doses. In reviewing the literature published up to the mid-1980s, the U.S. Environmental Protection Agency (EPA) concluded that blood lead levels in the range of 50–70 µg/dL are associated with an IQ decrement of approximately 5 points, blood lead levels of 30–50 µg/dL with a decrement of about 4 points, and blood lead levels of 15–30 µg/dL with a decrement of 1–2 IQ points (U.S. EPA, 1986). Since the mid-1980s, the results of a large number of additional cross-sectional and prospective studies were reported, providing the raw material for several meta-analyses designed to characterize general trends in the findings (e.g., Needleman & Gatsonis, 1990; Schwartz, 1994; World Health Organization, in press). In the World Health Organization (WHO) analysis, the regression coefficients describing the association between blood lead level and full-scale IQ obtained in 10 cross-sectional studies conducted in nine European countries were combined. Coefficients were weighted by the inverse of their variances to adjust for differences in sample sizes. The weighted common effect estimate was a decline of 2.1 IQ points for an increase from 10 µg/dL to 20 µg/dL (95% confidence interval: −1.2 to −3.1, $p < .001$). A similar analysis of the results of four prospective studies yielded a weighted estimate of −2.0 IQ points (95% confidence interval: −0.3 to −3.6, $p < .01$) for the relationship between mean postnatal blood lead level and school-age full-scale IQ. The WHO Task Group conducting this analysis concluded, "Based on the evidence from . . . populations with blood lead levels generally below 25 µg/dL, the size of the apparent IQ effect (at age 4 and above) is a deficit between 0 and 5 points (on a scale with a standard deviation of 15) for each 10 µg/dL increment in blood lead level, with a likely apparent effect size of between 1 and 3 [IQ] points. At blood lead levels above 25 µg/dL, the relationship between blood lead level and IQ may differ." The Task Group also concluded that "below the range of 10 to 15 µg/dL, the effect of confounding variables and limits in the precision of analytical and psychometric measurements increases the uncertainty attached to any estimate of effect. However, there is some evidence of an association below this range" (WHO, in press).

The consistency in results from different studies is much more striking for IQ than it is for scores on tests of specific neuropsychological domains (Bellinger, 1995b). To date, no specific cluster of functional deficits has been identified that can be considered to be the "behavioral signature" of lead. Many explanations for this can be offered. Most recent studies have focused on children with rather low lead burdens, near the presumed "threshold" of effect (or at least the threshold of detection), so that any deficits are subtle and most likely identifiable only with tests having the strongest psychometric characteristics (i.e., IQ tests). It may be necessary to study children with higher lead burdens (and thus more prominent deficits) in order to identify specific areas of weaknesses in neuropsychological function (e.g.,

Bellinger, Hu, Titlebaum, & Needleman, 1994). Another type of explanation focuses on the possibility that there may not be a single "signature" that is expressed in all children under all circumstances. Instead, the specific form of expression may depend on aspects of the "dosing regimen" such as timing (as a proxy for developmental stage), chronicity, and magnitude (e.g., Burdette & Goldstein, 1986; Dolinsky, Burright, & Donovick, 1983; Rice, 1992b; Shaheen, 1984). A third class of explanation rests on the assumption that the form in which toxicity is expressed varies with host and environmental characteristics such as genotype, rearing history, exposure and assessment settings, comorbidities, and coexposures (Bellinger, 1995a).

ACADEMIC ACHIEVEMENT AND "LEARNING DISABILITIES"

The lack of systematic research on the impact of different levels of lead intoxication on children's academic performance is surprising. Older, primarily clinic-based studies provide dramatic but anecdotal evidence that academic prognosis is poor for children with exposures sufficient to bring them to medical attention (Byers & Lord, 1943; de la Burde & Choate, 1975). In an 11-year follow-up of 132 of 270 children initially evaluated as first- and second-grade students, Needleman, Schell, Bellinger, Leviton, and Allred (1990) found that asymptomatic children with somewhat high lead levels in the dentin of shed deciduous teeth (>20 μg/g) were at significantly higher risk of failing to complete their secondary school program than were children with lead levels less than 10 μg/g (adjusted odds ratio, 7.4; 95% confidence interval, 1.4–40.7). They were also at greater risk of achieving reading scores two or more grades below the expected level (adjusted odds ratio, 5.8; 95% confidence interval, 1.7–19.7). A similar finding was reported in a study of a cohort of about 200 Danish second graders (Lyngbye, Hansen, Trillingsgaard, Beese, & Grandjean, 1990). The adjusted odds ratio for parent-reported learning disability associated with "high" circumpulpal dentin lead levels (>18.7 μg/g in one tooth or an arithmetic mean >16.0 μg/g for levels in two teeth) varied from 2.2 to 4.3, depending on the logistical regression model used. In this study, children with dentin lead levels less than 5 μg/g served as the reference group.

The evidence from cross-sectional studies is mixed with regard to whether the risk of academic dysfunction is increased among children with more modest elevations of lead burden (generally <30 μg/dL). Inverse relationships between lead burden and reading (primarily word reading) scores have been reported in some studies (Fergusson, Fergusson, Horwood, & Kinzett, 1988; Fergusson, Horwood, & Lynskey,

1993; Fulton et al., 1987; Yule, Lansdown, Millar, & Urbanowicz, 1981), although others have reported the absence of a statistically significant relationship (Ernhart, Landa, & Schell, 1981; Lansdown, Yule, Urbanowicz, & Hunter, 1986; Silva, Hughes, Williams, & Faed, 1988; Smith, Delves, Lansdown, Clayton, & Graham, 1983). Similarly, some studies have reported significant inverse relationships between lead and mathematics scores (Fergusson et al., 1988; Fulton et al., 1987), whereas others have not (Lansdown et al., 1986; Smith et al., 1983; Yule et al., 1981). In the only prospective study to report on academic achievement at school age, Bellinger, Stiles, and Needleman (1992) found an inverse relationship between children's battery composite scores on the Kaufman Test of Educational Achievement (K-TEA) (Brief Form) (Kaufman & Kaufman, 1985) at age 10 years and lead level measured at 2 years of age (a decline of 8.9 points per 10-µg/dL increase in blood lead). At this age, 90% of the children in the cohort had blood lead levels less than 13 µg/dL. The association was somewhat stronger for the mathematics and spelling subscales of the K-TEA than for the reading subscale.

Lead-associated elevations in pure-tone hearing threshold at various frequencies within the range of human speech have been reported among 4,519 4- to 19-year-old participants in the National Health and Nutrition Examination Survey II (NHANES II) (Schwartz & Otto, 1987) and among 3,262 6- to 19-year-old participants in the Hispanic Health and Nutrition Examination Survey (HHANES) (Schwartz & Otto, 1991). The estimated magnitude of pure-tone hearing loss was 1 dB for an increase in blood lead from 2 µg/dL to 10 µg/dL (Schwartz, 1993). Dietrich, Succop, Berger, and Keith (1992) presented additional evidence from the Cincinnati prospective lead study that neonatal and postnatal blood lead levels may impair central auditory processing of speech at age 5 years. These findings provide a plausible mechanism by which an increased lead burden might impede a child's learning.

PSYCHIATRIC AND BEHAVIORAL DISORDERS

The association between increased lead exposure and psychiatric and behavioral disorders in children has not been the topic of much empirical investigation. Although several case series and case-control studies suggested that children diagnosed as having autism tend to have higher blood lead levels (Accardo, Whitman, Caul, & Rolfe, 1988; Campbell et al., 1980; Cohen, Johnson, & Caparulo, 1976), the etiologic significance of this observation is not clear. Alternatively, aberrant behaviors that are part of the clinical presentation of children with autism (e.g., pica) may produce a secondary accumulation of lead.

Increased risk of secondary lead exposure has been described in psychotic children (McCracken, 1987; Oliver, 1967); children who were abused (Bithoney, Vandeven, & Ryan, 1993); children found to have aural, nasal, gastrointestinal, or foreign bodies (Wiley, Henretig, & Selbst, 1992); and children who are considered to be "accident prone" (Bond & Mathieu, 1992).

Because hyperactivity is reported to be a sequela of clinical lead poisoning (Chisolm, 1979), the hypothesis that "subclinical" lead poisoning is also a risk factor has received considerable attention. David and colleagues (David, Clark, & Voeller, 1972; David, Hoffman, Sverd, & Clark, 1977) claimed that hyperactive children whose medical histories did not include a "highly likely" cause for this disorder had higher blood lead levels and higher urine lead levels following a challenge dose of d-penicillamine. In a study similar in design, Gittelman and Eskenazi (1983) failed to find higher lead levels in a large group of cross-situationally hyperactive children than in a group of control children. However, a higher proportion of the hyperactive children had urinary lead levels greater than 0.8 mg/L (p = .06). In addition, hyperactive children had significantly higher urinary lead levels than their siblings. Unlike David and colleagues, Gittelman and Eskenazi (1983) did not find higher lead levels among hyperactive children with perinatal histories that were negative for complications.

The studies reviewed above leave considerable uncertainty about whether a child's risk of being diagnosed as hyperactive increases as the lead burden increases. In many recent epidemiologic studies, increased blood or tooth lead levels have been associated with teachers' ratings of children's hyperactivity using the Connors (1969) and Rutter (1967) rating scales (Fergusson et al., 1988, 1993; Silva et al., 1988; Thomson, et al., 1989; Yule, Urbanowicz, Lansdown, & Millar, 1984). However, direct observations of children's activity in naturalistic or laboratory settings have failed to reveal consistent associations with lead burden (Bellinger, Needleman, Bromfield, & Mintz, 1984; Hansen, Trillingsgaard, Beese, Lyngbye, & Grandjean, 1989; Harvey, Hamlin, & Kumar, 1984; Milar, Schroeder, Mushak, & Boone, 1981).

Several studies have reported associations between increased lead levels and many of the behavioral features of attention deficit hyperactivity disorder (e.g., distractibility, impulsivity, impersistence, inability to follow directions, daydreaming, low tolerance for frustration) (Hatzakis et al., 1985; Needleman et al., 1979; Yule et al., 1984). In other studies, however, this link has not been found (Bellinger et al., 1984; Winneke, Brockhaus, Ewers, Kramer, & Neuf, 1990). Positive associations have also been reported between blood lead level and teacher-reported "acting-out" behaviors. In a study of 501 Scottish children

6–9 years old with a mean blood lead level of 10.4 μg/dL, higher blood lead levels were associated with worse scores on the aggressive/antisocial subscale of the Rutter (1967) teacher scale, but not on the anxiety/neurotic subscale (Thomson et al., 1989). Similar results were reported on a sample of 166 6- to 12-year-old English children with a mean blood lead of 13.5 μg/dL (Yule et al., 1984) and in a study of 2- to 5-year-olds with blood lead levels persistently above 15 μg/dL (Sciarillo, Alexander, & Farrell, 1992). In a 1994 population-based study of behavior problems in a cohort of more than 1,250 8-year-olds, the prevalence of teacher-reported "internalizing" behaviors, as well as "externalizing" or acting-out behaviors, was associated with increased dentin lead levels (mean of 3.4 μg/g), but not with umbilical cord blood lead levels (mean of 6.8 μg/dL) (Bellinger, Leviton, Allred, & Rabinowitz, 1994). Among 493 Taiwanese, however, no association was found between tooth lead level (sample mean of 4.5 μg/g) and teacher-reported neurotic or antisocial behaviors (Rabinowitz, Wang, & Soong, 1993). The bases for these conflicting findings remain to be identified.

REVERSIBILITY

The seemingly straightforward question of whether cognitive effects associated with lead exposure are transient or enduring turns out not to yield a straightforward answer. This is attributable to several factors, including the lack of a commonly agreed-on operational definition of *reversibility*, the difficulty of finding tests of comparable psychometric characteristics suitable for assessing a specific cognitive domain longitudinally (reducing the likelihood of a measurement artifact), the ubiquity of some exposure to lead during each stage of the life span, and aspects of lead toxicokinetics (particularly the likelihood of endogenous inputs to blood lead even in the absence of external exposure) (Bellinger & Dietrich, in press). It can be difficult to ascertain whether any neurobehavioral deficits observed on follow-up assessment are maintained over time by ongoing exposure or by the gradual reequilibration of internal lead stores. It is important to recognize the possibility of a distinction between a "practical" and a "true" reversibility of lead-associated deficits (U.S. EPA, 1986).

Despite the complexities of this question, however, a number of follow-up studies provide data that may be useful to the clinician who wishes to estimate the developmental prognosis for a lead-exposed child. In the following section, the results of selected studies of children with varying levels of prior lead exposure are presented to illustrate the likelihood of recovery as a function of presumed dose.

The long-term outcome of children with severe lead poisoning was investigated by White, Diamond, Proctor, Morey, and Hu (1993). Thirty-four children treated between 1930 and 1942 at Children's Hospital (Boston) for clinical lead poisoning diagnosed before 4 years of age were followed up after 50 years. Their neuropsychological performances were compared with those of 20 controls matched for age, sex, race, and neighborhood. Blood lead levels were not available for these patients, although in all cases the medical record referred to clinical signs that are consistent with blood lead levels in excess of 60 μg/dL (e.g., abdominal pain, constipation, vomiting, anorexia, hyperirritability). The subjects with a history of poisoning performed worse on almost all of the tests administered, which covered the domains of IQ, memory, attention, visuomotor tracking, verbal fluency, nonverbal reasoning, motor speed, and mood. The authors suggested that the pattern of deficits indicated particular weaknesses in attention and executive functioning, reasoning, and short-term memory. Although the patients were similar to controls in terms of educational achievement, their occupational status was significantly lower. The authors concluded that "these findings are consistent with the hypothesis that many of the exposed subjects had acute encephalopathy in childhood that resolved into a chronic subclinical encephalopathy with cognitive dysfunction still evident in adulthood" (White et al., 1993, p. 620).

Benetou-Marantidou, Nakou, and Micheloyannis (1988) studied 30 6- to 11-year-old children who had always lived within 2 km of a primary lead smelter in Greece, comparing them to less exposed children matched on age, sex, family size, and socioeconomic and educational status of the parents. The exposed children had blood lead levels of 35–60 μg/dL. Neurobehavioral status was evaluated, in an unblinded manner, using the Rutter scale for parents (Rutter, Graham, & Yule, 1970), a standard neurologic examination, and the Oseretsky test for motor maturation. In addition, 23 of the exposed children and their matched controls (new matches in some cases) were followed up 4 years later using the Rutter questionnaire, a neurologic examination, and an assessment of school performance. Upon initial evaluation, the exposed group showed more abnormal findings on the neurologic examination (e.g., hypotonia, increased tendon reflexes, dysarthria, dysdiadochokinesia), poorer gross and fine motor function, and higher (more disturbed) scores on the Rutter questionnaire, especially the minimal brain dysfunction scale. Many of these differences were still evident 4 years later. In addition, only 2 of 23 exposed children were judged to be performing well at school (versus 11 of 23 controls). The authors concluded that "our findings constitute evidence of organic neurological dysfunction, which is persistent and may be irreversible, and also accounts for deficits in classroom performance" (Benetou-Marantidou et al., 1988, p. 395).

An 11-year follow-up study of children with elevated but subclinical dentin lead levels was reported by Needleman et al. (1990). Although blood lead levels were not measured as part of the initial phase of this study, the range was most likely approximately 15–50 µg/dL. In the evaluation conducted when the children were first and second graders, elevated dentin lead level was associated with a mild IQ deficit (approximately 4 points), lower performance on selected tests of language processing and attention, and less favorable teacher ratings of classroom performance (Needleman et al., 1979). Upon follow-up in late adolescence, children with elevated dentin lead levels performed worse on some (but not all) neuropsychological tests, including vocabulary, grammatical reasoning, hand–eye coordination, reaction time, and finger tapping. Their school performance was also worse: They had a lower mean class rank, greater absenteeism, poorer word-reading scores, and an increased risk of failing to complete their secondary school program. A third follow-up assessment, conducted at the age of 19–20 years, identified specific dimensions of attention as especially problematic for these children—namely, the ability to select and respond to target information and to shift focus adaptively (Bellinger, Hu, et al., 1994). As in the study by White et al. (1993), this pattern suggested that "executive" functions may be especially vulnerable to lead toxicity.

In a prospective study, Bellinger et al. (1992) described the results of assessments at age 10 years of a cohort of children followed since birth. At 5 years of age, higher levels of blood lead at age 2 years (in the range 0–25 µg/dL; 90th percentile: 13 µg/dL) were associated with lower general cognitive index scores on the McCarthy Scales of Children's Abilities (McCarthy, 1972) (Bellinger et al., 1991). This inverse association persisted over the next 5 years, as full-scale IQ at age 10 years was inversely associated with blood lead level at age 2 years (5.8 IQ point decline per 10-µg/dL increase). The mean blood lead level in this cohort at age 10 years was less than 3 µg/dL, making it unlikely that the deficits were maintained by recent exposure.

The data from these studies, which in aggregate involve children whose lead burdens cover a broad spectrum of exposures, suggest that lead-associated cognitive deficits may endure. The severity of the deficits appears to vary with exposure level, but even the subtle performance differences associated with the very modest elevations of blood lead in the cohort studied by Bellinger and colleagues (Bellinger et al., 1992) were detectable years later. These data are broadly consistent with those from primate studies (Davis, Otto, Weil, & Grant, 1990). Nevertheless, it is important to recognize that "persistent effects may not necessarily be permanent effects" (Davis et al., 1990, p. 219). Indeed, early developmental effects in children associated with elevations of increased prenatal exposure (i.e., <25 µg/dL) appear to be transient (Bellinger, Leviton, & Sloman, 1990; Bellinger, Leviton, Waternaux, Needleman, & Rabinowitz, 1987; Bellinger et al., 1991; Dietrich et al., 1987, 1990).

Little effort has been devoted to modeling temporal aspects of the relationship between early lead exposure and later performance. Fergusson and Horwood (1993) examined scores achieved annually between 8 and 12 years of age on the Burt Word Reading Test (Gilmore, Croft, & Reid, 1981) by 636 New Zealand children. Growth curve modeling techniques were used to compare the relative fit of three models to the association between dentin lead level and word-reading score: constant decrement, catch-up, and deterioration. At 8 years of age, children with dentin lead levels greater than 8 ppm achieved scores over the next 4 years that were consistently 4–6 months behind those of children with levels less than 3 ppm. The endurance of the initial setback in reading scores is thus consistent with the simple constant decrement model.

Meager information is available to help answer the question of whether medical treatment of lead-poisoned children prevents or reverses cognitive sequelae (Mortensen & Walson, 1993). Data from animal studies are not encouraging. Using a rodent model of the standard 5-day regimen of therapeutic chelation with calcium ethylenediaminetetraacetic acid (Ca EDTA), Cory-Slechta and Weiss (1989) found that treated rats continued to show the increased frequency of short interresponse times on a fixed interval schedule of food reinforcement that is typical of lead-exposed rats. Other studies from this lab suggest that a dosing regimen comparable to the Ca EDTA provocative chelation test produced increased brain lead levels (Cory-Slechta, Weiss, & Cox, 1987). Although brain levels were reduced by further administrations of Ca EDTA, 5 days of treatment did not produce any net loss in brain lead. The doses uses in these studies are higher, on a body weight basis, than those used in clinical treatment protocols, although Cory-Slechta and Weiss (1989) argue that they are similar on the basis of body surface area and basal metabolic equivalent. These data led some to advocate abandoning the lead mobilization test as a clinical procedure (Chisolm, 1987).

Several older studies of the sequelae of chelation therapy suggested that lead-poisoned children showed improved cognitive performance after chelation (Pueschel, Kopito, & Schwachman, 1972), or performed similarly to matched lower lead controls (Albert et al., 1974) or to presumably nonpoisoned siblings (Krall et al., 1980; Sachs et al., 1978). In a series of quasi-experimental studies of hyperactive children with blood lead levels that averaged 35 µg/dL, David et al. (David, Hoffman, Clark, & Sverd, 1983; David, Hoffman, Sverd, Clark, & Voeller, 1976; David, Katz, Arcoleo, & Clark, 1985) reported that administration of d-penicillamine produced significant behavioral improvement, but only among those children whose hyperactivity was judged to be of unknown origin. The authors speculated that a treatment effect was seen because the hyperactive behaviors of these children were maintained by an elevated body lead burden. This set of studies, though intriguing, suffers from a variety of methodologic problems, including ascertainment bias, poor characterization of exposure history, and weak statistical analysis (U.S. EPA, 1986).

Kirkconnell and Hicks (1980) reported that chelation failed to prevent a group of 22 lead-poisoned children (blood lead ≥50 µg/dL with erythrocyte protoporphyrin >110 on two successive occasions) from scoring significantly worse 4.5 months post-treatment than matched controls on the fine motor–adaptive subtest of the Denver Developmental Screening Test (Frankenburg, Camp, & Van Natta, 1971). However, the two groups of children achieved similar scores on the gross motor, personal–social, and language subtests.

The study design that would produce the most rigorous assessment of the efficacy of chelation therapy, a double-blind randomized clinical trial, has not been employed to date, although such a study is currently underway. A nonrandomized treatment trial of 154 13- to 87-month-old children with baseline blood lead levels between 25 µg/dL and 55 µg/dL suggested that any intervention that lowered blood lead, whether administration of Ca EDTA, iron supplementation, or source abatement, was associated with improved cognitive test performance 6 months post-treatment (Ruff, Bijur, Markowitz, Ma, & Rosen, 1993). The magnitude of this apparent effect, an increase of 1 point in cognitive score for each 3 µg/dL decrease in blood lead, is similar to the estimated magnitude of the association found between blood lead level and IQ in observational studies.

CONCLUSIONS

Extensive experimental research on animal cognition and on the cellular and subcellular neurotoxicity of lead provides a solid empirical basis for inferring that lead plays a causal role in the association noted in dozens of epidemiologic studies between increased lead burden and neurobehavioral deficits. Nevertheless, many issues remain unresolved. As Silbergeld (1992) observed, no underlying and unifying neurobiological mechanism of this effect has been identified to date, although many plausible candidates are under study (Pounds et al.,

1993). Similarly, the neuropsychological mechanisms underlying the performance effects remain to be explicated. Stollery, Broadbent, Banks, and Lee (1991) questioned whether lead produces a general impairment of cognition, produces independent impairments in several cognitive domains, or specifically targets a few key domains that underlie performance in many different domains. Current data provide little guidance in choosing one hypothesis over the others. Although the practical irreversibility of cognitive effects is supported by several studies, the reversibility of these effects on the mechanistic levels of analysis remains uncertain.

Considerable work is needed to clarify the likelihood that children with elevated lead burdens are at increased risk of psychiatric disorders. Like many other developmental diseases, lead poisoning is associated with a variety of poverty-related factors that place a child at increased risk for these disorders. Whether the increased risk observed among lead-exposed children reflects a causal or an epiphenomenal association is not yet clear. It does appear, however, that lead-poisoned children do not present a unique constellation of neuropsychological deficits. No particular sign or symptom has sufficient sensitivity, in the technical sense applied to medical screening tests, to alert the clinician to consider lead poisoning in the differential diagnosis. The neuropsychologist is thus unlikely to be the first clinician to identify a child as lead poisoned and is more likely to be called on for aid in characterizing and managing any neuropsychological problems associated with poisoning.

Considerably more is now known about the neuropsychological effects of lead poisoning than was known in the 1970s. Because much of the work done within this period was motivated largely by public health concerns, IQ usually served as the major neurobehavioral end point. The answers provided by these studies were sufficiently clear to justify dramatic revisions in public health and environmental policy. These, in turn, produced a startlingly large decline in community exposures to lead (Pirkle et al., 1994) and motivated the implementation of more aggressive identification and medical treatment strategies (Centers for Disease Control, 1991). Nevertheless, many important questions about the neuropsychological toxicity of lead remain unanswered (Bellinger, 1995a, 1995b).

REFERENCES

Accardo, P., Whitman, B., Caul, J., & Rolfe, U. (1988). Autism and plumbism: A possible association. *Clinical Pediatrics, 27,* 41–44.

Albert, R., Shore, R., Sayers, A., Strehlow, C., Kneip, T., Pasternack, B., Friedhoff, A., Covan, F., & Cimino, J. (1974). Follow-up of children overexposed to lead. *Environmental Health Perspectives, 7,* 33–39.

Bellinger, D. (1995a). Interpreting the literature on lead and child development: The neglected role of the "experimental system." *Neurotoxicology and Teratology, 17,* 201–212.

Bellinger, D. (1995b). Lead and neuropsychologic function in children: Progress and problems in establishing brain–behavior relationships. In M. Tramontana & S. Hooper (Eds.), *Advances in child neuropsychology* (Vol. 3, pp. 12–47). New York: Springer-Verlag.

Bellinger, D., & Dietrich, K. (in press). Recent studies of lead and neurobehavioral development in children. *Occupational Medicine: State of the Art Reviews.*

Bellinger, D., Hu, H., Titlebaum, L., & Needleman, H. (1994). Attentional correlates of dentin and bone lead levels in adolescents. *Archives of Environmental Health, 49,* 98–105.

Bellinger, D., Leviton, A., Allred, E., & Rabinowitz, M. (1994). Pre- and postnatal lead exposure and behavior problems in school-aged children. *Environmental Research, 66,* 12–30.

Bellinger, D., Leviton, A., & Sloman, J. (1990). Antecedents and correlates of improved cognitive performance in children exposed in utero to low levels of lead. *Environmental Health Perspectives, 89,* 5–11.

Bellinger, D., Leviton, A., Waternaux, C., Needleman, H., & Rabinowitz, M. (1987). Longitudinal analyses of prenatal and postnatal lead exposure and early cognitive development. *New England Journal of Medicine, 316,* 1037–1043.

Bellinger, D., Needleman, H., Bromfield, R., & Mintz, M. (1984). A follow-up study of the academic attainment and classroom behavior of children with elevated dentine lead levels. *Biological Trace Element Research, 6,* 207–223.

Bellinger, D., Sloman, J., Leviton, A., Rabinowitz, M., Needleman, H., & Waternaux, C. (1991). Low-level lead exposure and children's cognitive function in the preschool years. *Pediatrics, 87,* 219–227.

Bellinger, D., & Stiles, K. (1993). Epidemiologic approaches to assessing the developmental toxicity of lead. *Neurotoxicology, 14,* 151–160.

Bellinger, D., Stiles, K., & Needleman, H. (1992). Low-level lead exposure, intelligence and academic achievement: A long-term follow-up study. *Pediatrics, 90,* 855–861.

Benetou-Marantidou, A., Nakou, S., & Micheloyannis, J. (1988). Neurobehavioral estimation of children with life-long increased lead exposure. *Archives of Environmental Health, 43,* 392–395.

Bernstein, J. (1994). Assessment of developmental toxicity: Neuropsychological batteries. *Environmental Health Perspectives, 102* (Suppl. 2), 141–144.

Bithoney, W., Vandeven, A., & Ryan, A. (1993). Elevated lead levels in reportedly abused children. *Journal of Pediatrics, 122,* 719–720.

Bond, M., & Mathieu, O. (1992). Lead ingestion in a pattern of repetitive injury. *Clinical Pediatrics, 31,* 360–363.

Burdette, L., & Goldstein, R. (1986). Long-term behavioral and electrophysiological changes associated with lead exposure at different stages of brain development in the rat. *Developmental Brain Research, 29,* 101–110.

Byers, R., & Lord, E. (1943). Late effects of lead poisoning on mental development. *American Journal of Diseases of Children, 66,* 471–494.

Campbell, M., Petti, T., Green, W., Cohen, I., Genieser, N., & David, R. (1980). Some physical parameters of young autistic children. *Journal of the American Academy of Child Psychiatry, 19,* 193–212.

Centers for Disease Control (CDC). (1991). *Preventing lead poisoning in young children: A statement by the Centers for Disease Control—October 1991.* Atlanta, GA: U.S. Department of Health and Human Services.

Chisolm, J. (1979). Increased lead absorption and lead poisoning (plumbism). In V. Vaughn, R. McKay, & R. Behrman (Eds.), *Nelson textbook of pediatrics* (11th ed., pp. 2025–2029). Philadelphia: W.B. Saunders.

Chisolm, J. (1987). Mobilization of lead by calcium disodium edetate: A reappraisal. *American Journal of Diseases of Children, 141,* 1256–1257.

Cohen, D., Johnson, W., & Caparulo, B. (1976). Pica and elevated blood lead level in autistic and atypical children. *American Journal of Diseases of Children, 130,* 47–48.

Connors, C.K. (1969). A teacher rating scale for use in drug studies with children. *American Journal of Psychiatry, 126,* 884–888.

Cory-Slechta, D., & Weiss, B. (1989). Efficacy of the chelating agent CaEDTA in reversing lead-induced changes in behavior. *Neurotoxicology, 10,* 685–698.

Cory-Slechta, D., Weiss, B., & Cox, C. (1987). Mobilization and redistribution of lead over the course of CaNa₂EDTA chelation therapy. *Journal of Pharmacology and Experimental Therapeutics, 243,* 804–813.

David, O., Clark, J., & Voeller, K. (1972). Lead and hyperactivity. *Lancet, 2,* 900–903.

David, O., Hoffman, S., Clark, J., & Sverd, J. (1983). The relationship of hyperactivity to moderately elevated lead levels. *Archives of Environmental Health, 38,* 341–346.

David, O., Hoffman, S., Sverd, J., & Clark, J. (1977). Lead and hyperactivity: Lead levels among hyperactive children. *Journal of Abnormal Child Psychology, 5,* 405–416.

David, O., Hoffman, S., Sverd, J., Clark, J., & Voeller, K. (1976). Lead and hyperactivity: Behavioral response to chelation—a pilot study. *American Journal of Psychiatry, 133,* 1155–1158.

David, O., Katz, S., Arcoleo, C., & Clark, J. (1985). Chelation therapy in children as treatment of sequelae in severe lead toxicity. *Archives of Environmental Health, 40,* 109–113.

Davis, J., Otto, D., Weil, D., & Grant, L. (1990). The comparative developmental neurotoxicity of lead in humans and animals. *Neurotoxicology and Teratology, 12,* 215–229.

de la Burde, B., & Choate, M. (1975). Early asymptomatic lead exposure and development at school age. *Journal of Pediatrics, 87,* 638–642.

Dietrich, K., Krafft, K., Bornschein, R., Hammond, P., Berger, O., Succop, P., & Bier, M. (1987). Low-level fetal lead exposure effect on neurobehavioral development in early infancy. *Pediatrics, 80,* 721–730.

Dietrich, K., Succop, P., Berger, O., & Keith, R. (1992). Lead exposure and the central auditory processing abilities and cognitive development of urban children: The Cincinnati lead study cohort at age 5 years. *Neurotoxicology and Teratology, 14,* 51–56.

Dietrich, K., Succop, P., Bornschein, R., Krafft, K., Berger, O., Hammond, P., & Buncher, R. (1990). Lead exposure and neurobehavioral development in later infancy. *Environmental Health Perspectives, 89,* 13–19.

Dolinsky, Z., Burright, R., & Donovick, P. (1983). Behavioral changes in mice following lead administration during several stages of development. *Physiology and Behavior, 30,* 583–589.

Ernhart, C., Landa, B., & Schell, N. (1981). Subclinical levels of lead and developmental deficit: A multivariate follow-up reassessment. *Pediatrics, 67,* 911–919.

Fergusson, D., Fergusson, J., Horwood, L., & Kinzett, N. (1988). A longitudinal study of dentine lead levels, intelligence, school performance, and behaviour. *Journal of Child Psychology and Psychiatry, 29,* 811–824.

Fergusson, D., & Horwood, L. (1993). The effects of lead levels on the growth of word recognition in middle childhood. *International Journal of Epidemiology, 22,* 891–897.

Fergusson, D., Horwood, L., & Lynskey, M. (1993). Early dentine lead levels and subsequent cognitive and behavioural development. *Journal of Child Psychology and Psychiatry, 34,* 215–227.

Flegal, A., & Smith, D. (1992). Current needs for increased accuracy and precision in measurements of low levels of lead in blood. *Environmental Research, 58,* 125–133.

Frankenburg, W.K., Camp, B.W., & Van Natta, P.A. (1971). Validity of the Denver Developmental Screening Test. *Child Development, 42,* 475–485.

Fulton, M., Raab, G., Thomson, G., Laxen, D., Hunter, R., & Hepburn, W. (1987). Influence of blood lead on the ability and attainment of children in Edinburgh. *Lancet, 1,* 1221–1226.

Gilmore, A., Croft, C., & Reid, N. (1981). *Burt Word Reading Test New Zealand Revision: Teacher's Manual.* Wellington, New Zealand: NZCER.

Gittelman, R., & Eskenazi, B. (1983). Lead and hyperactivity revisited: An investigation of nondisadvantaged children. *Archives of General Psychiatry, 40,* 827–833.

Hansen, O., Trillingsgaard, A., Beese, I., Lyngbye, T., & Grandjean, P. (1989). A neuropsychological study of children with elevated dentine lead level: Assessment of the effect of lead in different socio-economic groups. *Neurotoxicology and Teratology, 11,* 205–213.

Harvey, P., Hamlin, M., & Kumar, R. (1984). Blood lead, behaviour and intelligence test performance in preschool children. *Science of the Total Environment, 40,* 45–60.

Hatzakis, A., Salaminios, F., Kokevi, A., Katsouyanni, K., Maravelias, K., Kalandidi, A., Koutselinis, A., Stefanis, K., & Trichopoulos, D. (1985). Blood lead and classroom behaviour of children in two communities with different degree of lead exposure: Evidence of a dose-related effect? In T.D. Lekkas (Ed.), *International Conference on Heavy Metals in the Environment* (Vol. 1, p. 47). Edinburgh, Scotland: CEP Consultants Ltd.

Kaufman, A., & Kaufman, N. (1985). *Kaufman Test of Educational Achievement–Brief Form Manual.* Circle Pines, MN: American Guidance Service.

Kirkconnell, S., & Hicks, L. (1980). Residual effects of lead poisoning on Denver Developmental Screening Test scores. *Journal of Abnormal Child Psychology, 8,* 257–267.

Krall, V., Sachs, H., Rayson, B., Lazar, B., Growe, G., & O'Connell, L. (1980). Effects of lead poisoning on cognitive performance. *Perceptual and Motor Skills, 50,* 483–486.

Lansdown, R., Yule, W., Urbanowicz, M., & Hunter, J. (1986). The relationship between blood-lead concentrations, intelligence, attainment and behaviour in a school population: The second London study. *International Archives of Occupational and Environmental Health, 57,* 225–235.

Lyngbye, T., Hansen, O., Trillingsgaard, A., Beese, I., & Grandjean, P. (1990). Learning disabilities in children: Significance of low-level lead-exposure and confounding factors. *Acta Paediatrica Scandinavia, 79*, 352–360.

McCarthy, D.A. (1972). *Manual for the McCarthy Scales of Children's Abilities*. New York: The Psychological Corporation.

McCracken, J. (1987). Lead intoxication psychosis in an adolescent. *Journal of the American Academy of Child and Adolescent Psychiatry, 26*, 274–276.

Milar, C., Schroeder, S., Mushak, P., & Boone, L. (1981). Failure to find hyperactivity in preschool children with moderately elevated lead burden. *Journal of Pediatric Psychology, 6*, 85–95.

Mortensen, M., & Walson, P. (1993). Chelation therapy for childhood lead poisoning: The changing scene in the 1990s. *Clinical Pediatrics, 32*, 284–291.

Needleman, H., & Gatsonis, C. (1990). Low-level lead exposure and the IQ of children: A meta-analysis of modern studies. *Journal of the American Medical Association, 263*, 673–678.

Needleman, H., Gunnoe, C., Leviton, A., Reed, R., Peresie, H., Maher, C., & Barrett, P. (1979). Deficits in psychologic and classroom performance of children with elevated dentine lead levels. *New England Journal of Medicine, 300*, 689–695.

Needleman, H., Schell, A., Bellinger, D., Leviton, A., & Allred, E. (1990). The long-term effects of exposure to low doses of lead in childhood: An 11-year follow-up report. *New England Journal of Medicine, 322*, 83–88.

Oliver, B. (1967). Aspects of lead absorption in hospitalised psychotic children. *Journal of Mental Deficiency Research, 11*, 132–142.

Pirkle, J., Brody, G., Gunter, E., Kramer, R., Paschal, D., Flegal, K., & Matte, T. (1994). The decline in blood lead levels in the United States: The National Health and Nutrition Examination Surveys (NHANES). *Journal of the American Medical Association, 272*, 284–291.

Pounds, J., Cory-Slechta, D., & Cranmer, J. (Eds.). (1993). New dimensions of lead neurotoxicity: Redefining mechanisms and effects [special issue]. *Neurotoxicology, 14*(2–3).

Pueschel, S., Kopito, L., & Schwachman, H. (1972). Children with an increased lead burden, a screening and follow-up study. *Journal of the American Medical Association, 222*, 462–466.

Rabinowitz, M., Wang, J.-D., & Soong, W.-T. (1993). Lead and classroom performance at seven primary schools in Taiwan. *Research in Human Capital and Development, 7*, 253–272.

Rice, D. (1992a). Behavioral impairment produced by developmental lead exposure: Evidence from primate research. In H. Needleman (Ed.), *Human lead exposure* (pp. 137–152). Boca Raton, FL: CRC Press.

Rice, D. (1992b). Lead exposure during different developmental periods produces different effects on FI performance in monkeys treated as juveniles and adults. *Neurotoxicology, 13*, 757–770.

Ruff, H., & Bijur, P. (1989). The effects of low to moderate lead levels on neurobehavioral functioning in children: Toward a conceptual model. *Journal of Developmental and Behavioral Pediatrics, 10*, 103–109.

Ruff, H., Bijur, P., Markowitz, M., Ma, Y-C., & Rosen, J. (1993). Declining blood lead levels and cognitive changes in moderately lead-poisoned children. *Journal of the American Medical Association, 269*, 1641–1646.

Rutter, M.A. (1967). A children's behavioral questionnaire for completion by teachers: Preliminary findings. *Journal of Child Psychology and Psychiatry, 8*, 1–11.

Sachs, H., Krall, V., McCaughran, D., Rozenfeld, I., Yongsmith, N., Growe, G., Lazar, B., Novar, L., O'Connell, L., & Rayson, B. (1978). IQ following treatment of lead poisoning: A patient–sibling comparison. *Journal of Pediatrics, 93*, 428–431.

Schwartz, J. (1993). Beyond LOEL's, p values, and vote counting: Methods for looking at the shapes and strengths of associations. *Neurotoxicology, 14*, 237–246.

Schwartz, J. (1994). Low level lead exposure and children's IQ: A meta-analysis and search for a threshold. *Environmental Research, 65*, 42–55.

Schwartz, J., & Otto, D. (1987). Blood lead, hearing thresholds, and neurobehavioral development in children and youth. *Archives of Environmental Health, 42*, 153–160.

Schwartz, J., & Otto, D. (1991). Lead and minor hearing impairment. *Archives of Environmental Health, 46*, 300–305.

Sciarillo, W., Alexander, G., & Farrell, K. (1992). Lead exposure and child behavior. *American Journal of Public Health, 82*, 1356–1360.

Shaheen, S. (1984). Neuromaturation and behavior development: The case of childhood lead poisoning. *Developmental Psychology, 20*, 542–550.

Silbergeld, E. (1992). Mechanisms of lead neurotoxicity, or looking beyond the lamppost. *FASEB Journal, 6*, 3201–3206.

Silva, P., Hughes, P., Williams, S., & Faed, J. (1988). Blood lead, intelligence, reading attainment and behaviour in eleven year old children in Dunedin, New Zealand. *Journal of Child Psychology and Psychiatry, 29*, 43–52.

Smith, M., Delves, T., Lansdown, R., Clayton, B., & Graham, P. (1983). The effects of lead exposure on urban children: The Institute of Child Health/Southampton study. *Developmental Medicine and Child Neurology, 25* (suppl. 47), 1–54.

Stollery, B., Broadbent, D., Banks, H., & Lee, W. (1991). Short-term prospective study of cognitive functioning in lead workers. *British Journal of Industrial Medicine, 48*, 739–749.

Thomson, G., Raab, G., Hepburn, W., Hunter, R., Fulton, M., & Laxen, D. -(1989). Blood-lead levels and children's behaviour: Results from the Edinburgh Lead Study. *Journal of Child Psychology and Psychiatry, 30*, 515–528.

U.S. Environmental Protection Agency (EPA). (1986). *Air quality criteria for lead*, EPA-600/08-83/028aF-dF (4 vols.). Research Triangle Park, NC: Author.

White, R., Diamond, R., Proctor, S., Morey, C., & Hu, H. (1993). Residual cognitive deficits 50 years after lead poisoning during childhood. *British Journal of Industrial Medicine, 50*, 613–622.

Wiley, J., Henretig, F., & Selbst, S. (1992). Blood lead levels in children with foreign bodies. *Pediatrics, 89*, 593–596.

Winneke, G., Brockhaus, A., Ewers, U., Kramer, U., & Neuf, M. (1990). Results from the European multicenter study on lead neurotoxicity in children: Implications for risk assessment. *Neurotoxicology and Teratology, 12*, 553–559.

World Health Organization (WHO). (in press). *IPCS Environmental Health Criteria for Inorganic Lead*. Geneva, Switzerland: Author.

Yule, W., Lansdown, R., Millar, I., & Urbanowicz, M. (1981). The relationship between blood lead concentrations, intelligence, and attainment in a school population: A pilot study. *Developmental Medicine and Child Neurology, 23,* 567–576.

Yule, W., Urbanowicz, M., Lansdown, R., & Millar, I. (1984). Teachers' ratings of children's behaviour in relation to blood lead levels. *British Journal of Developmental Psychology, 2,* 295–305.

7

LOW-LEVEL LEAD EXPOSURE DURING PREGNANCY AND ITS CONSEQUENCES FOR FETAL AND CHILD DEVELOPMENT

Kim N. Dietrich

O n the fate of the lead-poisoned conceptus . . .

> *It is generally agreed that if pregnancy does occur it is frequently charac-terized by miscarriage, intrauterine death of the fetus, premature birth and, if living children are born, they are usually smaller, weaker, slower in development and have a higher infant mortality.* (Cantarow & Trumper, 1944, p. 85)

Lead crosses the placenta readily and accumulates in fetal organs over the period of gestation (Barltrop & Burland, 1969; Mayer-Popken, Denkhaus, & Konietzko, 1986). The transplacental passage of lead is thought to take place by diffusion and is linearly related to the rate of umbilical blood flow (Goyer, 1990). The correlation between lead con-centrations in maternal and neonatal blood sampled at delivery can be quite high (e.g., >.80), especially in populations of women and neonates with high and variable exposures (Graziano et al., 1990;

This work was supported in part by a grant and contract from the National Insti-tute of Environmental Health Sciences, National Institutes of Health, U.S. Public Health Service.

McMichael, Vimpani, Robertson, Baghurst, & Clark, 1986). Although several of the physiologic changes that occur during pregnancy (e.g., hemodilution) would predict a substantial decline in blood lead over the course of gestation, studies have shown either a very slight decline in gravid maternal blood lead concentrations or relative stability from one trimester to another (Alexander & Delves, 1981). This equilibrium over the course of pregnancy is believed to be due to the continuous resorption of lead in deep physiologic depots such as the maternal skeleton (Silbergeld, 1991).

Lead has been recognized as an embryofetal poison since the turn of the 20th century. Women employed in lead enterprises at that time were observed to have much higher than expected rates of subfecundity, spontaneous abortion, and perinatal mortality. Oliver, a physician at the turn of the 20th century, made the grim observation that "when women worked in the white lead factories of Newcastle, they maintained that childbearing relieved them of the risks of becoming lead poisoned for they passed on the lead to the fetus in utero. The infant died, but the mother's body had parted with lead" (Oliver, 1914, p. 180).

The adverse reproductive and developmental consequences of high maternal blood lead concentrations during pregnancy are well documented and undisputed. In addition to Cantarow and Trumper's (1944) observations cited at the beginning of this chapter, more recent case studies of children whose mothers were lead poisoned during pregnancy corroborate earlier assessments. Such children have been found to be born preterm and growth retarded (Ghafour, Khuffash, Ibrahim, & Reavey, 1984; Palmisano, Sneed, & Cassady, 1969; Timpo, Amin, Casalino, & Yuceoglu, 1979). Furthermore, neurodevelopmental examination of these children during the neonatal and postnatal periods has demonstrated signs of significant prenatal central nervous system damage (Ghafour et al., 1984; Palmisano et al., 1969; Sensirivatana, Supachadhiwong, Phancharoen, & Mitrakul, 1983).

Because there is little serious debate concerning the reproductive and developmental consequences of congenital lead poisoning at higher levels (e.g., maternal blood lead concentrations in excess of 50 µg/dL), this chapter focuses primarily on the more unsettled question of intrauterine lead exposure at low to moderate doses and its potential effects on fetal and child development.

ENVIRONMENTAL CHEMICAL TERATOGENESIS

Careless industrial practices as well as industrial accidents have historically resulted in environmental pollution and contamination of human diets, with sometimes disastrous consequences for fetuses and postnatal survivors. For example, methyl mercury and organochlorine contamination of the diets of pregnant women in Asia and the Middle East resulted in intrauterine deaths, physical malformations, and developmental disabilities in postnatal survivors (Rogan, 1986; Weiss & Doherty, 1986). The pregnant women in some of these outbreaks were asymptomatic or presented with only minor symptoms at the same time that considerable damage to the conceptus occurred. Thus, by studying these tragic episodes, environmental toxicologists became sensitized to the fact that embryofetal toxicity was a possibility even in the absence of maternal signs or symptoms of poisoning.

Because more than 600 exogenous agents are known to produce teratogenic effects in animal laboratory experiments, it may come as a surprise to some that there are only two environmental chemicals listed as human teratogens in the seventh edition of Shephard's authoritative *Catalog of Teratogenic Agents*. Not surprisingly, the two chemicals Shephard lists are methyl mercury (MeHg) and the chloro-biphenyls, a class of synthetic compounds (Shephard, 1992). Lead does not appear among the listed human teratogenic agents, probably because it has never been associated with a specific cluster of major or minor malformations in humans. For example, Needleman and co-workers observed a significantly increased risk of minor congenital anomalies in a study of over 4,000 newborns with higher cord blood lead levels (Needleman, Rabinowitz, Leviton, Linn, & Schoenbaum, 1984). Newborns with umbilical cord blood lead concentrations great-er than 15 µg/dL were approximately two times more likely to present with a minor malformation. However, no specific pattern of malfor-mations was present among the various minor anomalies noted (e.g., hydrocele, hemangioma, lymphangioma, undescended testicles, vari-ous minor anomalies of the skin). Two other studies with much small-er sample sizes failed to replicate these results (Ernhart et al., 1986; McMichael et al., 1986).

Nevertheless, as previously mentioned, lead is a known abortifa-cient and the offspring of women working in the lead industries at the turn of the 20th century were sometimes reported to have low birth weight, microcephaly, mental handicap, and a high infant mortality (Oliver, 1914). Chronic fetal exposure to lead at moderate doses has also been implicated in the etiology of mild mental retardation (Beattie et al., 1975). Thus, if we expand the definition of a teratogenic chemi-cal to include substances capable of producing growth retardation and functional deficits, lead would appear to qualify as a human teratogen (Wilson, 1973). Indeed, in the 1992 revision of the *Catalog of Terato-genic Agents*, lead is listed as at least a "suspected teratogen," largely on the basis of some of the data reported by the international prospective studies of lead and child development (Shephard, 1992). The results of these investigations are summarized in the following pages.

This review is not exhaustive, because the literature is too vast to cover in a single chapter. Furthermore, the important but still quite unsettled question of the contribution of paternal lead exposure to embryofetal development is beyond the scope of this chapter (Sallmen, Lindbohm, Anttila, Taskinen, & Hemminiki, 1992). Instead, a representative sample of studies examining the relationship between indices of prenatal lead exposure and reproductive/developmental outcomes is presented.

ENVIRONMENTAL AND PHYSIOLOGIC SOURCES

With the virtual elimination of lead from gasoline in the United States, the atmosphere is now a minor source of lead exposure for most pregnant women. Exceptions would be women residing near point sources, such as primary or secondary smelters, or women working in an industry with inadequate emission controls and using lead in the manufacture of its products. Of course, women living in countries where alkyl lead is still added to motor fuels continue to be exposed to relatively high atmospheric concentrations.

Some hobbies may pose a risk as well, such as the fabrication of stained glass, bullets, or jewelry. Pregnant women who are involved in the rehabilitation of an older dwelling are also potentially at risk for respiration of lead particles or vapor if leaded paint is being sanded or flame stripped from the building's exterior or interior surfaces.

For most women today, diet is the principal source of nonoccupational exposure to lead. In the United States and some other developed countries, measures have been taken to reduce lead emissions over agricultural areas and eliminate lead solder from cans, resulting in a dramatic drop in the amount of lead in raw and processed foods since the late 1970s (World Health Organization, in press). However, imported foods in lead-soldered cans and foods prepared in imported glazeware are still a source of concern. Women in homes with lead plumbing and a soft water supply also are potentially at risk.

Consumption of tobacco and alcohol can be factors as well. Women who smoke have higher blood lead concentrations than nonsmokers (Ernhart, Wolf, Sokol, Brittenham, & Erhard, 1985). The consumption of spirits produced by domestic stills has been associated with dangerously high blood lead concentrations during pregnancy (Palmisano et al., 1969). The use of lead-containing folk remedies by Hispanic, Arabic, South Asian, and Hmong communities has been known to be a factor in prenatal exposure, as has the use of lead as a cosmetic by women from the Near East and South Asia (Flattery et al., 1993; Trotter, 1990). Women should also be cautious in the use of calcium supplements such as dolomite and bone meal powders, which have been shown to contain a significant amount of lead (Bourgoin, Evans, Cornett, Lingard, & Quattrone, 1993).

Under some circumstances, embryofetal lead burden cannot be estimated solely on the basis of the pregnant woman's gestational exposure. Because lead is stored principally in the skeleton, where it has a half-life measured in decades, there remains a possibility of embryofetal toxicity in the absence of any significant intake by the expectant mother. Some of the same hormonal processes that mobilize calcium during pregnancy and lactation also result in resorption of lead stored in bone. Thus, the accumulation of lead stored in a woman's skeleton prior to conception can be a potentially important contributing factor in the total dose to the conceptus (Silbergeld, 1991).

The notion that a woman's previous stores of lead play a role in total dose to the fetus has found support in some studies. For example, in analyses of data collected in the second National Health and Nutrition Examination Survey, it was reported that average blood lead levels were significantly higher in women who were beyond menopause. Moreover, the influence of menopause was smaller in women who had ever been pregnant. The authors of the study suggested that the stores of lead in the bones of these women had been partly depleted by pregnancy, thus leaving a lesser pool to be mobilized by the bone demineralization that accompanies the hormonal changes of menopause (Silbergeld, Schwartz, & Mahaffey, 1988). In an intriguing case study, the lead poisoning of a woman and her 11-month-old infant was described (Thompson, Robertson, & Fitzgerald, 1985). The woman, who was breastfeeding at the time, presented with a blood lead concentration of 75 µg/dL, whereas her infant's blood lead was measured at >50 µg/dL. The authors reported that there was no evidence of current environmental exposure over and above background levels in Australia. The woman's reproductive history was significant for several spontaneous abortions. Interestingly, the woman had been severely lead poisoned at the age of 18 months. It was speculated that pregnancy- and lactation-related hormonal alterations affecting calcium biokinetics had resulted in the resorption of large stores of lead from the maternal skeleton that had been acquired in childhood. This was then passed on to the fetus transplacentally and to the infant via breastfeeding.

Not much is known about how pregnancy affects previously acquired stores of lead. Many factors are likely to influence how much lead is released, including aspects of the mother's health (e.g., metabolic imbalances), maternal age, and prenatal nutrition. The role of maternal bone lead stores in fetal exposure may be clarified in the future as researchers attempt to employ methods such as K- and L-line X-ray fluorescence to assess changes in skeletal lead concentrations over the course of pregnancy (Rosen et al., 1993).

Early postnatal exposure to lead via breast milk is unlikely to be of concern, except in the case of women exposed to high levels of lead in occupational settings or other unusual circumstances (Ryu, Ziegler, & Fomon, 1978). Surveys of non–occupationally exposed lactating women have reported relatively low levels of lead in human milk, due in part to reductions in the concentration of lead in the atmosphere and diet (Rabinowitz, Leviton, & Needleman, 1985).

REPRODUCTIVE AND DEVELOPMENTAL CONSEQUENCES

Obstetric Complications and the Status of the Neonate

The evidence for adverse effects of maternal blood lead levels in the range of 1 µg/dL to approximately 30 µg/dL during the course of pregnancy on the health of the newborn is inconsistent. A study of pregnant women residing in areas proximal to heavy mining operations found that higher maternal and cord blood lead concentrations were significantly associated with premature rupture of the membranes and preterm birth (Fahim, Fahim, & Hall, 1976). For example, women closest to areas of mining activity who gave birth to preterm, low birth weight neonates had an average blood lead concentration at delivery of 29 µg/dL compared to a mean blood lead concentration of 14.3 µg/dL for women who delivered infants at term, with normal birth weights (Fahim et al., 1976).

Another group of investigators examined lead concentrations in human placentas from 1,971 normal and malformed deliveries in Birmingham, England (Wibberly, Khera, Edwards, & Rushton, 1977). In only 7% of the normal deliveries were placental lead levels greater than 1.5 µg/g; however, 61% of the neonatal deaths or stillbirths had higher concentrations of placental lead. Wibberly et al. (1977) caution that this does not necessarily implicate lead as a causal factor in fetal mortality. The authors offer the alternative explanation that lead accumulates in times of fetal stress. The lack of association between the concentration of lead in placenta and the cause of death would seem to support such an interpretation. The highest concentration of lead was found in the stillborn delivery of three infants with diagnoses of trisomy 18, ring D chromosome, and congenital cerebral tumor, respectively. The results of a similar and more recent study of pregnant women living near a long-standing lead smelter are also supportive of this view (Baghurst et al., 1991). Placental membrane samples obtained from stillbirths had, on average, 3.5 times higher concentrations of lead than those taken from normal births, and samples from preterm deliveries were 60% higher. However, the authors observed a very weak and nonsignificant correlation between maternal blood lead level at delivery and placental lead ($r = .08$), suggesting that factors additional to the pregnant woman's exposure to environmental lead were operative (Baghurst et al., 1991). What these other factors may be remains a matter of conjecture.

Several attempts have been made to assess less extreme reproductive and developmental outcomes of lead-exposed pregnancies. A number of international prospective studies have attempted to correlate low to moderate lead exposure with the gestational maturity and weight and stature of the newborn.

In Cincinnati, a significant association between prenatal maternal blood lead concentrations in the range of 1–27 µg/dL and birth weight was reported in 265 deliveries (Dietrich et al., 1987). In regression analyses controlling for other statistically significant factors including gestational age, number of prenatal visits, maternal stature, and cigarette, marijuana, and alcohol consumption, each µg/dL increment in prenatal blood lead was associated with a 20-g drop in weight at birth. This association is presented graphically in Figure 1.

However, the prospective studies have not been consistent in reporting lead's effects on fetal growth and maturation. The largest of these studies was conducted in Port Pirie, Australia, where emissions from a long-standing primary smelter resulted in widespread contamination of the surrounding environs (McMichael et al., 1986). A significant dose-dependent relationship was observed between maternal blood lead concentrations and the gestational maturity of the newborn in the case of 749 deliveries. Compared with women with blood lead concentrations of 8 µg/dL or less, the highest exposure group ($M = 17.1$ µg/dL) had a 4.4-fold increase in risk of preterm delivery after adjustment for maternal cofactors. However, no statistically significant associations were observed for birth weight or head circumference following adjustment for covariates (McMichael et al., 1986).

A prospective study of lead exposure and child development in the valley of Mexico City reported on the relationship between maternal prenatal and umbilical cord blood concentrations and head circumference measurements made in the first 2 years. Data from 111 deliveries were available. Maternal and cord blood lead concentrations were all below 37 µg/dL. After adjustment for covariates, higher mater-

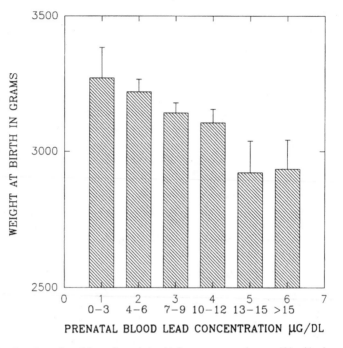

Figure 1.   Covariate-adjusted dose–effect relationship between maternal prenatal blood lead concentration measured in the first trimester of pregnancy and birth weight for 265 Cincinnati newborn infants. (Data originally reported in Dietrich et al., 1987.)

nal and cord blood lead concentrations were significantly associated with smaller head circumference at 6 and 18 months, respectively (Rothenberg et al., 1993).

A study of 4,354 pregnancies in Boston where the mean cord blood lead level was 7.0 ± 3.3 µg/dL found weak statistical evidence of an increased risk of delivery of a small-for-gestational-age newborn at concentrations above 15 µg/dL. The relationship between cord blood lead level and birth weight was negative but nonsignificant, and, contrary to the study's hypothesis, higher cord blood lead concentrations were significantly associated with increased gestational ages (Bellinger, Leviton, Rabinowitz, Allred, Needleman, & Schoenbaum, 1991).

Other prospective studies have not observed a significant association between prenatal lead exposure and measures of fetal development. A study conducted in Kosovo Province of the former Yugoslavia failed to observe any evidence of lead-related reductions in birth weight in over 900 deliveries (Factor-Litvak et al., 1991). This was the case despite the fact that many women in the study had blood lead concentrations in excess of 25 µg/dL. In a prospective study of fetal alcohol and lead exposure conducted in Cleveland, Ohio, no significant effects of low to moderate lead exposure on birth weight, head circumference, or length were reported (Ernhart et al., 1986).

Data from the prospective studies as well as others fail to provide a clear picture of the reproductive risks of low-to-moderate lead exposure, at least in terms of associations with intrauterine growth and maturation. There may be interactions involving nutritional, genetic, and other factors taking place in these studies that could make effects more apparent in one sample than another. In fact, the studies differ a great deal in terms of the ethnic and socioeconomic characteristics of their samples. Whatever effects on fetal growth and maturation may be present, they are small and apparently difficult to detect, even with large sample sizes.

Neurodevelopmental Consequences

The central nervous system (CNS) and neurobehavioral function are now regarded as the critical organ and critical effect, respectively, of lead. Inverse associations between lead exposure and behavioral development have defined the lowest acceptable doses when the risks of exposure have been under consideration by official advisory and regulatory bodies (Centers for Disease Control, 1991; World Health Organization, in press).

There are a number of potential mechanisms whereby lead may disrupt the development of the CNS in utero as well as during the early postnatal period. At very high doses, changes in the permeability of the vasculature of the brain result in the clinical picture of encephalopathy with cerebral and cerebellar edema as well as actual loss of neurons in the gray matter and gliosis (Goyer, 1982).

However, changes in vascular morphology are not evident with low-level lead exposure. Nevertheless, owing to the vulnerability of the immature blood–brain barrier, the fetal brain begins to accumulate lead at very low internal doses. This raises the question of whether lead has more subtle effects on CNS development (Goldstein, Asbury, & Diamond, 1974).

At low doses, it seems probable that lead perturbs processes such as synaptogenesis and other related neurodevelopmental phenomena that determine the finer structural properties of the brain (Averill & Needleman, 1980). Such effects would be neuropathologically occult, but may be detectable in the form of functional neurobehavioral deficits.

Evidence that lead at low or moderate doses can disturb CNS development is found in a growing number of in vitro and whole-animal studies. Research suggests that lead-related biochemical changes in the release of neurotransmitter substances could potentially disturb developmental processes involved in synaptic organization and function (Goldstein, 1990). Even at very low doses, lead has been demonstrated to have an antimitotic action, induce precocious growth of the neuroglia, and impair embryonic-to-adult conversion of the neural cell adhesion molecule. These represent processes that are intimately involved in the orchestration of brain histogenesis (Cookman, Hemmens, Keane, King, & Regan, 1988; Cookman, King, & Regan, 1987; Regan, Cookman, Keane, King, & Hemmens, 1989; Stark, Wolff, & Korbmacher, 1992).

Neurobehavioral Development

Compared to the number of epidemiologic studies of the neurobehavioral effects of postnatal lead exposure on children, relatively few investigators have attempted to determine if lead is developmentally neurotoxic in humans at low doses in utero. The reader should recall that, in most instances, *low dose* is defined in this chapter as a gravid maternal, cord, or neonatal blood lead concentration below 30 μg/dL.

At the present time, the best data available on this issue come from the international prospective studies conducted in Australia (Port Pirie and Sydney), Mexico (Mexico City), the United States (Boston, Cincinnati, and Cleveland), Scotland (Glasgow), and the former Yugoslavia (Kosovo Province). As of this writing, only pilot neurobehavioral data have been reported for the Mexico City prospective study (Rothenberg et al., 1989).

There were various sources of lead exposure for pregnant women at these sites, including lead-painted older dwellings (United States), fallout from long-standing primary smelters (Port Pirie and Kosovo), drinking water (Glasgow), and a complex mixture of environmental and dietary sources (Mexico City).

For a number of methodologic reasons, these forward studies are especially valuable in assessing the impact of lower-level prenatal lead exposure on child development. First, all of these investigations had quality control programs for the analysis of lead concentrations in blood samples from the mother, umbilical cord, and/or neonate. Analytic precision is critical in such studies, where many blood lead concentrations are low and restricted in range. Second, lead exposure was measured before or shortly following birth, rendering assertions about "reverse causality" moot (e.g., that, owing to intrinsic factors or other variables unrelated to lead, less intelligent youngsters are likely to ingest more soil and other lead-laden substances). Third, most studies had programs in place to ensure the quality of the neurobehavioral data that were collected. Furthermore, in meetings held prior to the beginning of data collection, the principal investigators arranged to use the same or similar measures of psychometric intelligence and behavior, thus permitting meaningful comparison of results across studies. Finally, potentially confounding factors were measured and included in multivariable data analyses (e.g., perinatal complications, maternal cigarette and alcohol consumption, social class, iron status, parental intelligence, quality of caregiving in the home environment).

In a series of papers published between 1984 and 1987, Bellinger and his colleagues at Children's Hospital in Boston implicated prenatal low-level lead exposure in the etiology of delays in sensorimotor and cognitive development measured repeatedly out to 2 years of age (Bellinger, Leviton, Needleman, Waternaux, & Rabinowitz, 1986; Bellinger, Leviton, Waternaux, Needleman, & Rabinowitz, 1987; Bellinger, Needleman, Leviton, Waternaux, Rabinowitz, & Nichols, 1984). Newborns were recruited on the basis of umbilical cord blood lead concentrations: low (<3 µg/dL), medium (6–7 µg/dL), and high (≥10 µg/dL). There were no cord blood lead concentrations in excess of 25 µg/dL. The Bayley Scales of Infant Development (Bayley, 1969) were employed to examine the cognitive and sensorimotor performance of approximately 249 children at 6, 12, 18, and 24 months of age.

The neurobehavioral effects of prenatal lead exposure observed in the Boston cohort were relatively small but statistically significant after adjustment for cofactors. Infants with cord blood lead concentrations below 3 µg/dL had average Bayley Mental Development Index scores about 5–8 points higher than infants with concentrations ≥10 µg/dL (Figure 2).

The Boston papers received widespread attention in the popular and scientific press. The study had an enormous impact on policies governing the regulation of lead in the environment and changed the standard of care for pediatric lead screening and treatment (Centers for Disease Control, 1991).

An unexpected repercussion of the Boston reports was the attempt by some industries to reinstate turn-of-the-century fetal protection policies designed to exclude women from the workplace (Bertin, 1994). In particular, the employment of women in the manufacture of lead acid batteries was contested (*International Union, UAW v. Johnson Controls,* 1991). The Supreme Court ultimately ruled that such policies violate Title VII of the Civil Rights Act of 1964 and the Pregnancy Discrimination Act of 1978 (Annas, 1991; Bertin, 1994).

In another follow-up of the Boston cohort at 5 and 10 years of age, significant associations between cord blood lead and measures of IQ and achievement were not observed (Bellinger, Sloman, Leviton, Rabinowitz, Needleman, & Waternaux, 1991; Bellinger, Stiles, & Needleman, 1992). However, children with higher postnatal blood lead concentrations evinced a slower rate of recovery than others in the cohort. Overall, these findings suggested that the early effects of low-

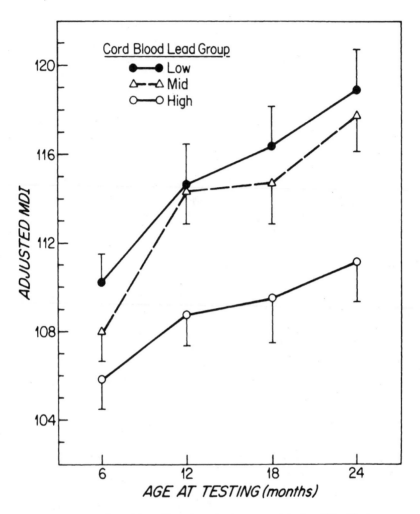

Figure 2.   Covariate-adjusted dose–effect relationship between umbilical cord blood lead concentrations and longitudinal Bayley Mental Development Index scores of infants in the Boston Prospective Study. Cord blood lead groups: low ≤3 μg/dL, medium 6–7 μg/dL, high ≥10 μg/dL. (From Bellinger, D., Leviton, A., Waternaux, C., Needleman, H., & Rabinowitz, M. [1987]. Longitudinal analyses of prenatal and postnatal lead exposure and early cognitive development. *New England Journal of Medicine, 316,* 1037; reprinted by permission.)

level fetal lead exposure are transient, an inference that is supported by the results of most other prospective studies.

   Some of the other international prospective studies have reported effects of fetal lead exposure on early postnatal development as well, but not with the internal consistency observed in the Boston data. In a birth cohort of over 300 infants in Cincinnati, a statistically significant inverse association was observed between prenatal maternal blood lead concentrations in the range of 1–27 µg/dL ($M = 8 \pm 3.7$ µg/dL) and the Mental and Psychomotor Development Index of the Bayley Scales at 3 and 6 months of age. Blood lead concentrations at 10 days of age were associated with lower Mental Index scores at 6 months. Significant interactions were also observed, with Mental Index scores of males and infants from the poorest families associated more strongly with perinatal blood lead concentrations. Further analyses employing structural equation modeling (a form of path analysis) suggested that a portion of the effect of prenatal lead exposure on development was mediated by lead's association with reduced birth weight and gestational maturity. When infants were evaluated 18 months later, statistically significant associations between Bayley Scale scores and perinatal blood lead were no longer evident (Dietrich et al., 1990). Subjects therefore appeared to have recovered from lead-related deficits in sensorimotor development assessed at 6 months. Indeed, further analyses of these data revealed that infants of mothers with the highest prenatal blood lead levels showed the greatest percent increase in Bayley Mental Development Index scores in four assessments conducted between 3 and 24 months. These findings were viewed as consistent with a hypothesis of neurobehavioral catch-up growth for infants whose CNS maturation may have been compromised by intrauterine lead exposure or other gestational factors that influenced prenatal growth and maturation (Dietrich et al., 1990).

When the Cincinnati cohort was examined at 4 years of age, higher neonatal blood lead concentrations were significantly associated with lower scores on subscales of Kaufman Assessment Battery for Children (Kaufman, 1983) (an assessment of information processing abilities, IQ, and academic achievement). This association was especially strong among children from the poorest families in the cohort (Dietrich, Succop, Berger, Hammond, & Bornschein, 1991). Further follow-up of these children with psychometric assessments at 5 and 6.5 years of age revealed no remaining statistically significant associations between indices of prenatal lead exposure and intellectual attainment after adjustment for covariates (Dietrich, Berger, Succop, Hammond, & Bornschein, 1993; Dietrich, Succop, Berger, & Keith, 1992). However, at 5 years of age, higher neonatal blood lead concentrations were associated with poorer performance on the Filtered Word subtest of the SCAN, a measure of central auditory processing skills (Dietrich et al., 1992). Furthermore, at 6 years of age, higher neonatal blood lead concentrations were significantly and inversely associated with the lower gross and fine motor coordination scale scores on the Bruininks–Oseretsky Test of Motor Proficiency (Bruininks, 1978) (Dietrich, Berger, & Succop, 1993). For the Cincinnati study at least, higher perinatal blood lead levels continued to be associated with developmental deficits in some areas of neurobehavioral development as late as 6 years of age.

In the prospective study conducted in Port Pirie, Australia, assessment of neurobehavioral developmental status did not commence until later infancy. Tests employed included the Bayley Scales at 2 years, the McCarthy Scales of Children's Abilities (McCarthy, 1972) at 4 years, and the revised Wechsler Intelligence Scale for Children (Wechsler, 1974) at 7 years. Prenatal maternal and umbilical cord blood lead concentrations averaged approximately 10 and 8 µg/dL, respectively.

Although postnatal blood lead levels were predictive of lower attainment, neither average antenatal nor cord blood lead concentrations were associated with scores on these exams following adjustment for potentially confounding variables such as measures of caregiver behavior and stimulation in the home, social class, and maternal intelligence. An intriguing aspect of the Port Pirie data is the enormous impact of covariate adjustment on study results. For example, for 4-year-old children, each log increment in antenatal average blood lead was associated with a statistically significant drop of 15 ± 4.7 IQ points (or 1 standard deviation) in the General Cognitive Index of the McCarthy Scales—a very large effect. Following adjustment for potential confounders, the decrement in the cognitive index score was reduced to a statistically nonsignificant 1.8 ± 5.7 points (McMichael et al., 1988).

The Port Pirie cohort was evaluated again at 7 years of age with the revised Wechsler Intelligence Scale for Children (Baghurst et al., 1992). Following covariate adjustment, none of the measures of prenatal exposure was significantly associated with Verbal, Performance, or Full Scale IQ.

Another prospective study in Australia was conducted in Sydney. This was a 7-year follow-up investigation of a birth cohort of over 300 children recruited from three metropolitan hospitals in 1983. The geometric means for maternal and cord blood lead concentrations were 9 and 8 µg/dL, respectively. The results of this prospective study are more easily abstracted than most. At no point in the study were significant inverse associations between perinatal blood lead concentrations and outcomes observed either prior to or following adjustment for covariates (Cooney, Bell, McBride, & Carter, 1989a, 1989b; Cooney, Bell, & Stavron, 1991).

A prospective investigation in Cleveland, Ohio, of the developmental consequences of prenatal maternal alcoholism included prenatal maternal and cord blood lead assessments as part of the study's protocol (Ernhart et al., 1985). Approximately 50% of the mothers were positive for alcohol abuse as assessed by the Michigan Alcoholism Screening Test (Selzer, 1971). Like the Cincinnati study, this was a sample of urban, lower socioeconomic status women and their children. Approximately 250 families were recruited for this study, but the number of subjects in any analysis involving blood Pb was often fewer than 200 because of missing data. Mean cord blood Pb for 162 samples was 5.8 µg/dL, whereas for 185 maternal blood samples obtained at delivery, it was 6.5 µg/dL. No perinatal blood leads exceeded 15 µg/dL (Ernhart et al., 1986).

Results of the Cleveland study have been mixed, and the investigators have always interpreted the overall nature of their findings as negative. At 1 day of age, neonates' scores on the Muscle Tonus and Soft Signs subscales of the Graham/Rosenblith Behavioral Examination for Newborns (Rosenblith, 1979) were significantly associated with cord and maternal blood lead concentration, respectively. The Abnormal Reflexes Cluster of the Brazelton Neonatal Behavioral Assessment Scale (Brazelton, 1973) was significantly associated with cord but not maternal blood lead level (Ernhart et al., 1986). Six months later statistically significant inverse associations between maternal blood lead and neurodevelopmental status were also observed on the Bayley Scales and the Kent Infant Development Scale (Reuter & Beckett, 1985) (Ernhart, Morrow-Tlucak, Marler, & Wolf, 1987). Continued follow-up of this cohort to approximately 5 years revealed no further relationships between perinatal blood lead levels and development following adjustment for covariates (Ernhart, Morrow-Tlucak, Wolf, Super, & Drotar, 1989).

The Cleveland study has engendered some controversy among lead researchers and other analysts. For example, it has been suggested that the decision to investigate within a single sample the independent and joint effects of lead and alcohol may have biased findings for both exposures toward failure to reject the null hypothesis (Bellinger & Needleman, 1994; Thacker, Hoffman, Smith, Steinberg, & Zack, 1994). In the design of epidemiologic studies of relatively weak associations, recruitment of a cohort free of other exposures likely to produce the disease under investigation is usually recommended (Rothman & Poole, 1988).

A prospective study in Glasgow (Moore, Bushnell, & Goldberg, 1989) evaluated 151 subjects developmentally at 12 and 24 months of age with the Bayley Scales of Infant Development (Bayley, 1969). The sample was divided into three groups on the basis of maternal prenatal blood lead concentration: high (>30 µg/dL), medium (15–25 µg/dL), and low (<10 µg/dL). Prior to as well as following adjustment for covariates, no statistically significant associations between maternal prenatal blood lead levels and Bayley scores were observed. Apparently, no further follow-up of this cohort has been attempted.

The prospective study conducted in Kosovo Province examined a birth cohort of approximately 300 children at 6, 12, 18, 24, 36, and 48 months of age (Wasserman et al., 1992, 1994). The study was conducted in two towns in the province—Mitrovica, the site of a lead smelter and battery plant, and Pristina, an area of lesser atmospheric pollution about 25 miles south of the lead industrial operations. This cohort differed from the other prospective studies in that over a third of the children were anemic during infancy (i.e., hemoglobin <10.5 g/dL at age 2 years). Prenatal maternal blood lead concentration averaged 19.9 ± 7.7 µg/dL in women residing in Mitrovica and 5.6+/−2.0 µg/dL for women in the "unexposed" region of Pristina. The Bayley Scales of Infant Development (1969) were employed to assess cognitive developmental status throughout infancy, and the McCarthy Scales of Children's Abilities were given to children at ages 3 and 4 years.

Even before adjusting for potential confounding variables, no statistically significant associations between any perinatal blood lead measure and 2-year Bayley Mental Development Index (1969) scores were observed. However, at 3 and 4 years of age and following adjustment for covariates, higher prenatal and cord blood lead concentrations were significantly associated with lower General Cognitive Index scores on the McCarthy Scales. Children's scores on subtests of the Perceptual Performance subscale were particularly affected. For example, on the Perceptual Performance subscale, which has a mean of 50 and standard deviation of 10, children of mothers with prenatal blood lead values greater than 20 µg/dL scored a full standard deviation below children in the lowest exposure group (<5 µg/dL prenatal blood lead).

The authors assert that their ability to detect associations between prenatal lead exposure and preschool psychometric intelligence may be due to the relatively wide range of fetal exposure in the Kosovo cohort. Indeed, among the international prospective studies, this is the most heavily exposed cohort prenatally. However, the authors also claim that the negative results of some of the other prospective studies, such as the one conducted in Cincinnati, are attributable to the "extreme social deprivation" of the sample, thus hampering detection of the more subtle associations with lead exposure (Wasserman et al., 1994). This is a puzzling interpretation coming from the authors of a positive study of undernourished children from a war-torn country. In any event, the Kosovo study strongly suggests that prenatal blood lead concentrations exceeding 20 µg/dL may present a long-term hazard to optimal intellectual development.

Except for the Cincinnati cohort, where an association was observed between low-level perinatal lead exposure and deficits in central auditory processing and gross and fine motor coordination (Dietrich et al., 1992, 1993a), the results of the prospective studies collectively imply that the effects of low-level fetal lead exposure on neurobehavioral development may be transient or limited to the varieties of sensorimotor behaviors assessed during infancy. The Kosovo study demonstrated a strong and robust relationship between prenatal lead exposure and preschool psychometric intelligence. However, it is apparent that many of the women in this study were exposed at levels more typical of the lead occupations. For example, 25% of the women in the study had integrated prenatal blood lead concentrations from midpregnancy to delivery of between 20 and 42 µg/dL (Wasserman et al., 1994). This undermines the generalizability of the Kosovo study's findings to the more widespread problem of general community lead exposure at lower levels. However, it suggests that women working in industries without adequate controls for employee exposure to lead may be subjecting their children to a risk for later cognitive deficits. The Kosovo study may resurrect once again the debate surrounding the employment of women with reproductive potential in industries using lead.

Although prenatal blood lead concentrations below 25 µg/dL do not appear to be associated with long-term deficits in cognitive development, this has not turned out to be the case for early postnatal lead exposure (see Chapter 6). Results of the international prospective studies indicate that postnatal blood lead concentrations greater than 10–20 µg/dL are associated with small but statistically significant declines in school-age IQ and measures of academic achievement (Baghurst et al., 1992; Bellinger et al., 1992; Dietrich et al., 1993b). The debate concerning the impact of lead exposure during the preschool years appears to be drawing to a close. Discussion is presently centered on the most cost-efficient means by which childhood lead exposure may be prevented or effectively treated.

CONCLUSIONS

The clinical picture of low-level fetal lead exposure appears to be one of mild growth retardation in utero (although the data are inconsistent in this regard) and mild developmental delay up to ages 1–2 years with recovery by school age or somewhat earlier.

The negative nature of the prospective neurobehavioral studies of older children should not encourage clinicians to ignore exposure of the fetus to lead as a potential threat to in utero and postnatal CNS development. Women need to be counseled to reduce or eliminate exposure to this developmentally neurotoxic metal both prior to and during pregnancy. The administration of drugs designed to enhance excretion of lead (chelators) during pregnancy is an extremely unattractive option because of the metabolic side effects of these drugs and because they have some teratogenic potential (Liebelt & Shannon, 1994). Primary prevention is the only reasonable strategy.

Finally, it must be stressed that the prospective studies reviewed in this chapter employed multiple regression methodologies that described statistical trends in large samples of children. It is probable that there is a great deal of interindividual variability in the sensitivity of fetuses to lead at low doses. It is unwise to assume that all children exposed to lead in utero will necessarily recover developmentally from earlier deficits in cognition and behavior.

REFERENCES

Alexander, F.W., & Delves, H.T. (1981). Blood lead levels during pregnancy. *International Archives of Occupational and Environmental Health, 48,* 35–39.

Annas, G.J. (1991). Fetal protection and employment discrimination: The *Johnson Controls* case. *New England Journal of Medicine, 49,* 204–205.

Averill, D.R., & Needleman, H.L. (1980). Neonatal lead exposure retards cortical synaptogenesis in the rat. In H.L. Needleman (Ed.), *Low level lead exposure and the clinical implications of the current research* (pp. 201–210). New York: Raven Press.

Baghurst, P.A., McMichael, A.J., Wigg, N.R., Vimpani, G.V., Robertson, E.F., Roberts, R.J., & Tong, S. (1992). Environmental exposure to lead and children's intelligence at the age of seven years: The Port Pirie Cohort Study. *New England Journal of Medicine, 327,* 1279–1284.

Baghurst, P.A., Robertson, E.F., Oldfield, R.K., King, B.M., McMichael, A.J., Vimpani, G.V., & Wigg, N.R. (1991). Lead in placenta, membranes, and umbilical cord in relation to pregnancy outcome in a lead-smelter community. *Environmental Health Perspectives, 90,* 315–320.

Barltrop, D., & Burland, W.L. (1969). *Mineral metabolism in pediatrics.* Philadelphia: F.A. Davis.

Bayley, N. (1969). *Bayley Scales of Infant Development: Birth to two years.* New York: The Psychological Corporation.

Beattie, A.D., Moore, M.R., Goldberg, A., Finlayson, M.J.W., Graham, J.F., Mackie, E.M., Main, J.C., McLaren, D.A., Murdoch, R.M., & Stewart, G.T. (1975). Role of chronic lead exposure in the aetiology of mental retardation. *Lancet, 1,* 589–591.

Bellinger, D.C., Leviton, A., Needleman, H.L., Waternaux, C., & Rabinowitz, M. (1986). Low-level lead exposure and infant development in the first year. *Neurotoxicology and Teratology, 8,* 151–161.

Bellinger, D., Leviton, A., Rabinowitz, M., Allred, E., Needleman, H., & Schoenbaum, S. (1991). Weight gain and maturity in fetuses exposed to low levels of lead. *Environmental Research, 54,* 151–158.

Bellinger, D., Leviton, A., Waternaux, C., Needleman, H., & Rabinowitz, M. (1987). Longitudinal analyses of prenatal and postnatal lead exposure and early cognitive development. *New England Journal of Medicine, 316,* 1037–1043.

Bellinger, D.C., & Needleman, H.L. (1994). The neurotoxicity of prenatal exposure to lead: Kinetics, mechanisms, and expressions. In H.L. Needleman & D.C. Bellinger (Eds.). *Prenatal exposure to toxicants: Developmental consequences.* Baltimore: Johns Hopkins University Press.

Bellinger, D.C., Needleman, H.L., Leviton, A., Waternaux, C., Rabinowitz, M.B., & Nichols, M.L. (1984). Early sensorimotor development and prenatal exposure to lead. *Neurotoxicology and Teratology, 6,* 387–402.

Bellinger, D., Sloman, J., Leviton, A., Rabinowitz, M., Needleman, H.L., & Waternaux, C. (1991). Low level lead exposure and children's cognitive function in the preschool years. *Pediatrics, 87,* 219–227.

Bellinger, D.C., Stiles, K.M., & Needleman, H.L. (1992). Low-level lead exposure, intelligence and academic achievement: A long-term follow-up study. *Pediatrics, 90,* 855–861.

Bertin, J.E. (1994). Reproductive hazards in the workplace: Lessons learned from *UAW v. Johnson Controls.* In H.L. Needleman & D. Bellinger (Eds.), *Prenatal exposure to toxicants: Developmental consequences* (pp. 297–316). Baltimore: Johns Hopkins University Press.

Bourgoin, B.P., Evans, D.R., Cornett, J.R., Lingard, S.M., & Quattrone, A.J. (1993). Lead content in 70 brands of dietary calcium supplements. *American Journal of Public Health, 83,* 1155–1160.

Brazelton, T.B. (1973). *Neonatal Behavioral Assessment Scales.* Philadelphia: J.B. Lippincott.

Bruininks, R.H. (1978). *The Bruininks-Oseretsky Test of Motor Proficiency.* Circle Pines, MN: American Guidance Service.

Cantarow, A., & Trumper, M. (1944). *Lead poisoning.* Baltimore: Williams & Wilkins.

Centers for Disease Control. (1991). *Preventing lead poisoning in young children: A statement by the Centers for Disease Control—October, 1991.* Washington, DC: U.S. Department of Health and Human Services, Public Health Service, Centers for Disease Control.

Cookman, G.R., Hemmens, S.E., Keane, G., King, W.B., & Regan, C.M. (1988). Chronic low level lead exposure precociously induces rate glial development in vitro and in vivo. *Neuroscience Letters, 86,* 33–37.

Cookman, G.R., King, W., & Regan, C.M. (1987). Chronic low-level lead exposure impairs embryonic to adult conversion of neural cell adhesion molecule. *Journal of Neurochemistry, 49,* 399–403.

Cooney, G.H., Bell, A., McBride, W., & Carter, C. (1989a). Low-level exposures to lead: The Sydney Lead Study. *Developmental Medicine and Child Neurology, 31,* 640–649.

Cooney, G.H., Bell, A., McBride, W., & Carter, C. (1989b). Neurobehavioral consequences of prenatal low level exposures to lead. *Neurotoxicology and Teratology, 11,* 95–104.

Cooney, G., Bell, A., & Stavron, C. (1991). Low level exposures to lead and neurobehavioral development: The Sydney study at seven years. In *Proceedings of the international conference on heavy metals in the environment* (Vol. 1). Edinburgh, Scotland: CEP Consultants Ltd.

Dietrich, K.N., Berger, O.G., & Succop, P.A. (1993a). Lead exposure and the motor developmental status of urban six-year-old children in the Cincinnati Prospective Study. *Pediatrics, 91,* 301–307.

Dietrich, K.N., Berger, O.G., Succop, P.A., Hammond, P.B., & Bornschein, R.L. (1993b). The developmental consequences of low to moderate prenatal and postnatal lead exposure: Intellectual attainment in the Cincinnati Lead Study cohort following school entry. *Neurotoxicology and Teratology, 15,* 37–44.

Dietrich, K.N., Krafft, K.M., Bornschein, R.L., Hammond, P.B., Berger, O., Succop, P.A., & Bier, M. (1987). Low-level fetal lead exposure effect on neurobehavioral development in early infancy. *Pediatrics, 80,* 721–730.

Dietrich, K.N., Succop, P.A., Berger, O.G., Hammond, P.B., & Bornschein, R.L. (1991). Lead exposure and the cognitive development of urban preschool children: The Cincinnati Lead Study cohort at age 4 years. *Neurotoxicology and Teratology, 13*, 203–211.

Dietrich, K.N., Succop, P.A., Berger, O.G., & Keith, R.W. (1992). Lead exposure and the central auditory processing abilities and cognitive development of urban children: The Cincinnati Lead Study cohort at age 5 years. *Neurotoxicology and Teratology, 14*, 51–56.

Dietrich, K.N., Succop, P.A., Bornschein, R.L., Krafft, K.M., Berger, O., Hammond, P.B., & Buncher, C.R. (1990). Lead exposure and neurobehavioral development in early infancy. *Environmental Health Perspectives, 89*, 13–19.

Ernhart, C.B., Morrow-Tlucak, M., Marler, M., & Wolf, A.W. (1987). Low level lead exposure in the prenatal and early preschool periods: Early preschool development. *Neurotoxicology and Teratology, 9*, 259–270.

Ernhart, C.B., Morrow-Tlucak, M., Wolf, A.W., Super, D., & Drotar, D. (1989). Low level lead exposure in the prenatal and early school periods: Intelligence prior to school entry. *Neurotoxicology and Teratology, 11*, 161–170.

Ernhart, C.B., Wolf, A.W., Kennard, M.J., Erhard, P., Filipovich, H.F., & Sokol, R.J. (1986). Intrauterine exposure to low levels of lead: The status of the neonate. *Archives of Environmental Health, 41*, 287–291.

Ernhart, C.B., Wolf, A.W., Sokol, R.J., Brittenham, G.M., & Erhard, P. (1985). Fetal lead exposure: Antenatal factors. *Environmental Research, 38*, 54–66.

Factor-Litvak, P., Graziano, J.H., Kline, J., Popovac, D., Mehmeti, A., Murphy, M.J., Gashi, E., & Haxhiui, R. (1991). A prospective study of birth weight and length of gestation in a population surrounding a lead smelter in Kosovo, Yugoslavia. *International Journal of Epidemiology, 20*, 722–728.

Fahim, M.S., Fahim, Z., & Hall, D.G. (1976). Effects of subtoxic lead levels on pregnant women in the state of Missouri. *Research Communications in Chemical Pathology and Pharmacology, 13*, 309–331.

Flattery, J., et al. (1993). Lead poisoning associated with use of traditional and ethnic remedies—California, 1991–1992. *Morbidity and Mortality Weekly Report, 42*(27), 521–524.

Ghafour, S., Khuffash, F., Ibrahim, H., & Reavey, P. (1984). Congenital lead intoxication with seizures due to prenatal exposure. *Clinical Pediatrics, 23*, 282–283.

Goldstein, G.W. (1990). Lead poisoning and brain cell function. *Environmental Health Perspectives, 89*, 91–94.

Goldstein, G.W., Asbury, A., & Diamond, I. (1974). Pathogenesis of lead encephalopathy. *Archives of Neurology, 31*, 382–389.

Goyer, R.A. (1982). Lead toxicity. In J.J. Chisolm & D.M. O'Hara (Eds.), *Lead absorption in children: Management, clinical and environmental aspects*. Baltimore: Urban & Schwarzenberg.

Goyer, R.A. (1990). Transplacental transfer of lead. *Environmental Health Perspectives, 89*, 101–105.

Graziano, J.H., Popovac, D., Factor-Litvak, P., Shrout, P., Kline, J., Murphy, M.J., Zhao, Y., Mehmeti, A., Ahmedi, X., Rajovic, B., Zvicer, Z., Nenezic, D., Lolacono, N.J., & Stein, Z. (1990). Determinants of elevated blood lead during pregnancy in a population surrounding a lead smelter in Kosovo, Yugoslavia. *Environmental Health Perspectives, 89*, 95–100.

International Union, UAW v. Johnson Controls, 499 U.S. 187, 111A S. Ct. 1196 (1991).

Kaufman, A.S. (1983). *Kaufman Assessment Battery for Children (K-ABC)*. Circle Pines, MN: American Guidance Service.

Liebelt, E., & Shannon, M.W. (1994). Oral chelators for childhood lead poisoning. *Pediatric Annals, 23*, 616–626.

Mayer-Popken, O., Denkhaus, W., & Konietzko, H. (1986). Lead content of fetal tissues after maternal intoxication. *Archives of Toxicology, 58*, 203–204.

McCarthy, D.A. (1972). *Manual for the McCarthy Scales of Children's Abilities*. New York: The Psychological Corporation.

McMichael, A.J., Baghurst, P.A., Wigg, N.R., Vimpani, G.V., Robertson, E.F., & Roberts, R.J. (1988). Port Pirie cohort study: Environmental exposure to lead and children's abilities at the age of four years. *New England Journal of Medicine, 319*, 468–475.

McMichael, A.J., Vimpani, G.V., Robertson, E.F., Baghurst, P.A., & Clark, P.D. (1986). The Port Pirie cohort study: Maternal blood lead and pregnancy outcome. *Journal of Epidemiology and Community Health, 40*, 18–25.

Moore, M.R., Bushnell, I.W.R., & Goldberg, Sir A. (1989). A prospective study of the results of changes in environmental lead exposure in children in Glasgow. In M.A. Smith, L.D. Grant, & A.I. Sors (Eds.), *Lead exposure and child development: An international assessment* (pp. 371–378). Dordrecht, the Netherlands: Kluwer Academic.

Needleman, H.L., Rabinowitz, M., Leviton, A., Linn, S., & Schoenbaum, S. (1984). The relationship between prenatal exposure to lead and congenital anomalies. *Journal of the American Medical Association, 251*, 2956–2959.

Oliver, T. (1914). *Lead poisoning from the industrial, medical, and social points of view*. Baltimore: Williams & Wilkins.

Palmisano, P.A., Sneed, R.C., & Cassady, G. (1969). Untaxed whiskey and fetal lead exposure. *Journal of Pediatrics, 75*, 869–872.

Rabinowitz, M., Leviton, A., & Needleman, H. (1985). Lead in milk and infant blood: A dose–response model. *Archives of Environmental Health, 40*, 283–286.

Regan, C.M., Cookman, G.R., Keane, G.J., King, W., & Hemmens, S.E. (1989). The effects of chronic low-level lead exposure on the early structuring of the central nervous system. In M.A. Smith, L.D. Grant, & A.I. Sors (Eds.), *Lead exposure and child development: An international assessment* (pp. 440–452). Dordrecht, the Netherlands: Kluwer Academic.

Reuter, J., & Beckett, L. (1985). *The Kent Infant Development Scale* (2nd ed.). Kent, OH: Kent Development Metrics, Inc.

Rogan, W.J. (1986). PCB's and cola colored babies: Japan, 1968, and Taiwan, 1979. In J.L. Sever & R.L. Brent (Eds.), *Teratogen update: Environmentally induced birth defects* (pp. 127–130). New York: Alan R. Liss.

Rosen, J.F., Crocetti, A.F., Balbi, K., Balbi, J., Bailey, C., Clemente, I., Redkey, N., & Grainger, S. (1993). Bone lead content assessed by L-Line fluorescence in lead-exposed and non-lead-exposed suburban populations in the United States. *Proceedings of the National Academy of Sciences, 90*, 2789–2792.

Rosenblith, J. (1979). The Graham/Rosenblith Behavioral Examination for Newborns: Prognostic value and procedural issues. In J.D. Osofsky (Ed.), *Handbook of infant development* (pp. 216–249). New York: John Wiley & Sons.

Rothenberg, S.J., Schnaas, L., Cansino-Ortiz, S., Perroni-Hernandez, E., De La Torre, P., Neri-Mendez, C., Ortega, P., Hidago-Loperena, H., & Svendsgaard,

D. (1989). Neurobehavioral deficits after low level lead exposure in neonates: The Mexico City Pilot Study. *Neurotoxicology and Teratology, 11*, 85–93.

Rothenberg, S.J., Schnaas-Arrieta, L., Perez-Guerrero, I.A., Perroni-Hernandez, E., Mercado-Torres, L., Gomez-Ruez, C., & Zea, F. (1993). Prenatal and postnatal blood lead level and head circumference in children to three years: Preliminary results from the Mexico Prospective Lead Study. *Journal of Exposure Analysis and Environmental Epidemiology, 3*, 165–172.

Rothman, K.J., & Poole, C. (1988). A strengthening programme for weak associations. *International Journal of Epidemiology, 17*, 955–959.

Ryu, J.E., Ziegler, E.E., & Fomon, S.J. (1978). Maternal lead exposure and blood lead concentration in infancy. *Journal of Pediatrics, 93*, 476–478.

Sallmen, M., Lindbohm, M., Anttila, A., Taskinen, H., & Hemminiki, K. (1992). Paternal occupational lead exposure and congenital malformations. *Journal of Epidemiology and Community Health, 46*, 519–522.

Selzer, M.L. (1971). The Michigan Alcoholism Screening Test. *American Journal of Psychiatry, 127*, 769–774.

Sensirivatana, R., Supachadhiwong, O., Phancharoen, S., & Mitrakul, C. (1983). Neonatal lead poisoning: An unusual clinical manifestation. *Clinical Pediatrics, 22*, 582–584.

Shephard, T.H. (1992). *Catalog of teratogenic agents* (7th ed.). Baltimore: The Johns Hopkins University Press.

Silbergeld, E.K. (1991). Lead in bone: Implications for toxicology during pregnancy and lactation. *Environmental Health Perspectives, 91*, 63–70.

Silbergeld, E.K., Schwartz, J., & Mahaffey, K. (1988). Lead and osteoporosis: Mobilization of lead from bone in postmenopausal women. *Environmental Research, 47*, 79–94.

Stark, M., Wolff, J.E.A., & Korbmacher, A. (1992). Modulation of glial cell differentiation by exposure to lead and cadmium. *Neurotoxicology and Teratology, 14*, 247–252.

Thacker, S.B., Hoffman, D.A., Smith, J., Steinberg, K., & Zack, M. (1994). Letter to the editor. *Archives of Environmental Health, 49*, 204–205.

Thompson, G.N., Robertson, E.F., & Fitzgerald, S. (1985). Lead mobilization during pregnancy. *Medical Journal of Australia, 143*, 131.

Timpo, A., Amin, J., Casalino, M., & Yuceoglu, A. (1979). Congenital lead intoxication. *Journal of Pediatrics, 94*, 765–767.

Trotter, R.T. (1990). The cultural parameters of lead poisoning: A medial anthropologist's view of intervention in environmental lead exposure. *Environmental Health Perspectives, 89*, 79–84.

Wasserman, G., Graziano, J.H., Factor-Litvak, P., Popovac, D., Morina, N., Musabegovic, A., Vrenezi, N., Capuni-Paracka, S., Lekic, V., Preteni-Redjepi, E., Hadzialjevic, S., Slavkovich, V., Kline, J., Shrout, P., & Stein, Z. (1992). Independent effects of lead exposure and iron deficiency anemia on developmental outcome at age 2 years. *Journal of Pediatrics, 121*, 695–703.

Wasserman, G.A., Graziano, J.H., Factor-Litvak, P., Popovak, D., Morina, N., Musabegovic, A., Vrenezi, N., Capuni-Paracka, S., Lekic, V., Preteni-Redjepi, E., Hadzialjevic, S., Slavkovich, V., Kline, J., Shrout, P., & Stein, Z. (1994). Consequences of lead exposure and iron supplementation on childhood development at age 4 years. *Neurotoxicology and Teratology, 16*, 233–240.

Wechsler, D. (1974). *Wechsler Intelligence Scale for Children—revised edition.* New York: The Psychological Corporation.

Weiss, B., & Doherty, R.A. (1986). Methylmercury poisoning. In J.L. Sever & R.L. Brent (Eds.), *Teratogen update: Environmentally induced birth defects* (pp. 119–121). New York: Alan R. Liss.

Wibberly, D.G., Khera, A.K., Edwards, J.H., & Rushton, D.I. (1977). Lead levels in human placentae from normal and malformed births. *Journal of Medical Genetics, 14,* 339–345.

Wilson, J.G. (1973). *Environment and birth defects.* New York: Academic Press.

World Health Organization (WHO). (in press). *IPCS Environmental Health Criteria for Inorganic Lead.* Geneva, Switzerland: Author.

8

MEDICAL MANAGEMENT

J. Julian Chisolm, Jr.

L ead poisoning is a chronic disease. The most important component of medical management is to facilitate reduction in the child's exposure to environmental lead. This overrides all other considerations. With the virtually complete removal of lead from gasoline and food, deteriorated lead paint in older housing is the major source of lead for children in the United States today (Pirkle et al., 1994). The Centers for Disease Control and Prevention (CDC) recommended in the 1991 guidelines (CDC, 1991a) that any child with a blood lead concentration (PbB)[1] ≥20 µg/dL whole blood be examined by a physician. Indeed, where available, such children should be referred to a lead treatment clinic where comprehensive management is most likely to be obtained. The team should include physicians, nurse practitioners, public health nurses, psychologists, and medical social workers and should maintain close liaison with public health workers in the local health department. It is the local health department that usually has the authority to require abatement of lead paint hazards in old houses. In many states, blood lead concentrations must be reported to a state or local governmental department by laboratories performing the analyses. The CDC recommends that all children be followed until at least 6 years of age. Those with disabilities may have to be followed for a much longer time, particularly if excessive hand-to-mouth activity or pica persists. Medical management at the very least includes monitor-

[1]All blood lead concentrations mentioned in this chapter refer to confirmed venous blood lead levels as measured in a laboratory proficient in such measurements.

ing of adequate nutrition, instruction in proper dust suppression, and identification of potential sources of lead. Clinical decisions should always be based on venous blood lead measurements. Control of exposure to lead is vitally important among toddlers because hand-to-mouth activity and pica are most prevalent and intense during this age period. Furthermore, current scientific evidence indicates that this is the time at which injury to the developing nervous system occurs, although any resulting learning disabilities may not become evident until school age. For example, effects on neurobehavioral and academic performance at 10 years of age are best predicted by blood lead concentration at 2 years of age (Bellinger, Stiles, & Needleman, 1992). For older children in whom excessive hand-to-mouth activity has stopped and serial blood lead values show a declining trend, major emphasis in management switches to the identification of neurobehavioral disabilities, which may require special educational management in school. In the 1990s, public health emphasis began to shift from treatment to prevention through reducing exposure. The CDC's strategic plan calls for elimination of childhood lead poisoning by the year 2010 (CDC, 1991b).

CLASSIFICATION OF BLOOD LEAD CONCENTRATIONS

The CDC recommends that the intensity of follow-up be based on several ranges in blood lead concentration (Table 1). Blood lead concentrations in Class I are currently considered acceptable. There is no further follow-up other than that required for screening. When the child's blood lead concentration falls within Classes IIA and IIB, it is recommended that the child be followed by the primary care provider, who should pay careful attention to the child's nutrition and to the cleaning techniques used in the home. The CDC recommends, however, that all children with blood lead concentrations ≥20 µg/dL whole blood (Classes III and IV) be examined by a physician. Such children should be referred to a lead treatment center, if available. Children

Table 1. Blood lead classification

Blood lead range (µg/dL whole blood)[a]	CDC class[b]
0–9	I
10–14	IIA
15–19	IIB
20–44	III
45–69	IV
≥70	V

[a]To convert to µmol/L, divide by 20.72.
[b]Adapted from CDC (1991a).

with blood lead concentrations ≥70 μg/dL whole blood (Class V) should be hospitalized immediately and treated as medical emergencies. In CDC Classes III and IV, children should be followed closely, with priority given to younger children with the higher blood lead levels (details are discussed below).

Absorption, Distribution, Storage, and Excretion of Lead

Lead is absorbed into the body through both the respiratory and gastrointestinal tracts. It also moves transplacentally to the fetus. Absorption through these different routes varies and is affected by age, nutritional status, particle size, and chemical form of the lead. Absorption is inversely proportional to particle size; this is a factor that makes lead-bearing dust so important. Adults absorb 6%–10% of dietary lead and retain very little of it; however, children from birth to 2 years of age have been shown to absorb 40%–50% and to retain 20%–25% of dietary lead. Spontaneous excretion of lead in urine by infants and young toddlers is normally about 1 μg/kg/24 hr, which may increase somewhat in acute poisoning. Dietary intake of lead is <1 μg/kg, which provides a margin of safety in the sense that a child goes into positive lead balance when intake exceeds 5 μg/kg of body weight (Ziegler, Edwards, Jensen, Mahaffey, & Fomon, 1978).

The body lead burden is divided into three main compartments—blood, soft tissue, and bone—with subcompartments in each of these (Rabinowitz, Wetherill, & Kopple, 1976). The average residence time of lead in blood is approximately 25 days. In soft tissues such as the liver and kidney, lead has an average residence time of about 40 days. The average residence time of lead in bone varies from about 3 years in trabecular bone to 30 years in cortical bone. There is thought to be a subcompartment in periosteal bone that may be more readily mobilized, as during chelation therapy. At least 70% of the total-body lead burden in children is found in bone. Lead can enter the body very quickly but is excreted from the body very slowly (see also Chapter 5).

Nutritional Factors

Studies in experimental animals have repeatedly shown that deficient dietary intakes of iron, zinc, copper, and calcium can enhance the absorption and toxicity of lead (Mahaffey, 1981). Sources that are adequate in iron are generally adequate also in zinc and copper. Studies in lead-poisoned rats show that iron deficiency anemia may not be fully correctable if the animal is copper deficient (Klander & Petering, 1977). This may be relevant to iron-deficient human infants with lead toxicity because nutritional iron deficiency in infants and toddlers is often associated with grossly excessive intakes of whole cow's milk, which is also deficient in copper. Dietary sources of iron include liver, ground beef, fortified cereal, cooked legumes, and spinach. It is important to ensure an adequate but not excessive intake of calcium. In both children and animals, dietary deficiencies of calcium enhance the absorption of lead (Ziegler et al., 1978). Experimental studies strongly indicate that interactions between lead and calcium play a highly significant role in the toxicity of lead (Goldstein, 1992). An adequate intake of calcium can be ensured by a maximum daily intake of 32 ounces of iron-fortified formula during the first 24 months of life. After that, an intake of 16–24 ounces of whole cow's milk is adequate. For children who are intolerant of whole cow's milk, yogurt, cheese, and calcium-fortified bread provide good alternative sources of calcium. If a child refuses whole cow's milk, sometimes chocolate or other flavor additives will make the milk acceptable to the child. Although not documented in humans, excessive intake of fat in experimental animals clearly enhances the absorption of lead. It is therefore considered prudent to trim excess obvious fat from meats and to remove skin and the adjacent fat from chicken.

In summary, the diet for a child with lead toxicity is simply a good diet with adequate protein and mineral intake and limitation of excess fat. It is no longer necessary to exclude canned foods and beverages when the cans are manufactured in the United States, as the manufacture of cans with lead-soldered seams ended in the United States in 1991[2] (Pirkle et al., 1994).

Dust Suppression

It is clear that there is a significant relationship between lead in paint and soil and the interior household dust, which in turn is significantly related to hand lead and then blood lead (Bornschein et al., 1986; Davies et al., 1990). It is therefore of great importance that dust lead be suppressed and that all surfaces that the child can touch, such as window sills, window wells, banisters, door jambs, and so forth, be cleaned using high-phosphate detergents such as automatic dishwasher detergents.[3] Depending on circumstances, these surfaces should probably be cleaned twice weekly. Also, children's hands and their toys should be washed frequently. Lead has been found in particulates not readily trapped by ordinary vacuum cleaners. Over the years in the author's clinic, medical social service workers have been invaluable in assisting families with their multiple and varied requirements. They

---

[2]The Food and Drug Administration is undertaking steps to control the importation of foods and beverages in cans with lead-soldered seams.

[3]Dilute 1 ounce of detergent containing 5% phosphorus in 1 gallon of water. Mop or damp-dust with this solution, changing solution frequently.

assist families in relocating to lead-safe housing and provide advice on sources of funding for housing repairs where available. The present deleading projects being sponsored by the U.S. Department of Housing and Urban Development should facilitate relocation of families to lead-safe housing in the coming years (see also Chapter 9).

Laboratory Tests for Iron Deficiency

Iron deficiency can enhance absorption and toxicity of lead and often coexists with overexposure to lead. All children with a blood lead concentration ≥ 20 µg/dL whole blood should have appropriate testing for iron deficiency (CDC, 1991a). Table 2 shows tests that are useful in the differential diagnosis of common forms of microcytosis. Lead poisoning, for example, does not produce microcytosis and anemia until the blood lead concentration rises well above 60 µg/dL whole blood. The erythrocyte protoporphyrin (EP) test does not readily discriminate between iron deficiency anemia and lead poisoning when the increase in blood lead concentration is moderate; however, extraordinary elevations in EP are encountered when iron deficiency anemia and severe lead poisoning occur together. There are two options: Give a therapeutic trial of iron or try to substantiate the diagnosis of iron deficiency by determining the serum iron (SI), total iron binding capacity (TIBC), and/or serum ferritin. Of course, these are more costly tests. Because serum iron may fluctuate (e.g., in relation to intercurrent infection), the SI/TIBC ratio is useful only if the TIBC is elevated. Serum ferritin can be falsely elevated in children with intercurrent illnesses. If a therapeutic trial of iron is chosen, an increase of 1.0 g/dL or more in hemoglobin concentration after a month may be considered diagnostic of iron deficiency anemia when iron (as ferrous sulfate) is given in a dose of 3 mg/kg of body weight per day. If such a response is observed, iron

Table 2.   Differential diagnosis of microcytosis

Index[a]	Iron deficiency	Heterozygous α- or β-thalassemia trait	Lead poisoning
Hemoglobin	Reduced	Reduced	Normal[b]
MCV	Reduced	Reduced	Normal[c]
FEP	Increased	Normal	Increased
Serum iron	Reduced	Normal	Normal
TIBC	Increased	Normal	Normal
Ferritin	Reduced	Normal	Normal

(Note that two or more of these conditions may coexist.)

From Oski, F. (1993). Iron deficiency in infancy and childhood. *New England Journal of Medicine, 329,* 192; reprinted by permission.

[a]MCV, mean corpuscular volume; FEP, free erythrocyte protoporphyrin; TIBC, total iron binding capacity.

[b]May be decreased if the blood lead concentration is in excess of 100 µg Pb/dL.

therapy should be continued for an additional 2–3 months. If such an increase is not observed, the therapeutic trial should be discontinued (Oski, 1993).

Erythrocyte Protoporphyrin

Elevation in EP indicates impairment in the biosynthesis of heme in the developing erythrocyte in the bone marrow. Heme is formed when iron is incorporated into protoporphyrin IX. In iron deficiency, the iron supply is insufficient and EP levels as zinc protoporphyrin (ZnPP) increase. Lead interferes with the utilization of iron for heme formation. In either case, excess protoporphyrin IX accumulates as ZnPP, a metalloporphyrin that is stable and remains in the red cell throughout its life span. In lead poisoning, there is usually a delay of 3–4 weeks before this effect in the bone marrow is reflected by an increase in the EP level in peripheral blood. EP is a sensitive screening test for iron deficiency (Hastka, Lasserre, Schwarz-beck, & Hehlmann, 1994). (See also Chapter 6.)

Use of Paired Blood Lead and
Erythrocyte Protoporphyrin Results in Medical Management

Although the EP test is not sufficiently sensitive to serve as a primary screening test for lead poisoning, serial EP values, together with serial PbB values, are extremely important in monitoring trends in this chronic disorder. EP, when elevated, reflects long-term trends in lead absorption. After effective medical and environmental interventions, both PbB and EP (if elevated) will decrease slowly over months or years, although not necessarily at the same rate (Chisolm, 1982). EP levels are particularly helpful in at least two situations:

1. Immediately after chelation, PbB virtually always increases by 5–10 µg/dL whole blood during the first 2–4 weeks. If at the same time EP, after 3–4 weeks, shows a decrease in comparison with the immediate postchelation value, it is most likely that there is internal redistribution of lead. However, when EP after 3–4 weeks shows a definite increase, the physician should strongly suspect that the patient has continued to ingest excess amounts of lead following chelation therapy. This, in turn, would trigger the physician to initiate a search for the source of lead.

2. Sometimes a significant increase in PbB following lower and apparently stable serial PbB measurements is encountered. Such a sharp increase raises the question of contamination of the sample as opposed to a real increase in PbB. If there has really been chronically increased lead absorption over a period of several weeks or months, EP will also increase, thus pointing to chronic excess

assimilation. However, it might be an isolated episode of excess lead ingestion shortly before the blood sample was obtained rather than a more chronic increase. In that case, EP will not show any change. In either case, PbB and EP should be repeated within 2–4 weeks.

Other Tests

The calcium disodium edetate ($CaNa_2EDTA$; EDTA = ethylenediaminetetraacetic acid) mobilization test for lead has in the past played a significant role in clinical investigation and is still used in some medical centers to select children with blood lead levels of 25–45 µg/dL whole blood on the basis that those with a positive test will respond to chelation therapy with a brisk diuresis of lead. However, studies have shown no long-term differences between those with negative and positive tests (Markowitz, Bijur, Ruff, & Rosen, 1993). It might further be noted that about 85% of children whose blood lead levels fall between 40 and 45 µg/dL whole blood are reported to have a positive mobilization test. Chelation should be considered in these children without performing a mobilization test. Because of the great difficulty in obtaining timed collections of urine in children under 3 years of age, this test is impractical and liable to give misleading information in the general pediatric situation. Radiologic tests are in general of limited usefulness. Radiographic examination of the abdomen is not necessary in most children. In the mid-1990s, most of the children identified with increased blood lead concentrations fall into CDC Classes IIA, IIB, and III (Table 1). In these children, the increase is most likely attributable to the repetitive ingestion of small particulate lead in dust and soil. Such particles are too small to be identified on a clinical X ray. If done, a clinical radiograph may show radiopaque material in the gut if that material has been ingested during the preceding 24–36 hours. Medical management is not likely to be influenced by radiographic findings unless a retained lead object (i.e., fishing weight) is found in the stomach. Radiographic examinations of bone will only show bands of increased density at the metaphyseal plates at the knee and wrist when blood lead levels are sustained for 6–12 weeks or longer at levels in excess of 50–60 µg/dL whole blood. These tests no longer play a significant role in the clinical management of lead poisoning. Basophilic stippling is not always found even in severe lead poisoning. It is not a useful diagnostic test; however, if basophilic stippling is found, it should prompt measurement of the blood lead level. Likewise, concentrations of lead in hair and fingernails do not correlate with blood lead levels. These tests are not useful in diagnosis, because they are confounded by external contamination.

In vivo X-ray fluorescence of lead in bone has been under development since the 1970s. Most studies have been conducted in adults. It is useful to measure long-term accumulation of lead because the residence time of lead in bone is so long. Its use so far has been restricted to clinical research studies. At present, it appears unlikely that in vivo measurement of lead in bone will replace any existing measurements of lead exposure. Rather, such measurements are likely in the future to supplement existing tests in order to gain information on lead pools that cannot otherwise be made except by biopsy. Whether in the future it will replace the provocative chelation test is unknown (Todd & Chettle, 1994).

EVALUATION AND FOLLOW-UP
FOR A CHILD WITH BLOOD LEAD ≥20 µg/dL
WHOLE BLOOD WHO IS NOT ON CHELATION THERAPY

Initial Visit

Medical management includes monitoring for adequate nutrition, repeated counseling in dust suppression, and tentative identification of probable environmental lead sources (see also Chapter 9). Initially, a confirmatory venous blood lead test is done. A detailed history is taken, including the presence or absence of clinical symptoms; the child's hand-to-mouth activity, including the existence of pica; nutritional status; iron, calcium, and fat intake; family history of lead poisoning; identification of potential sources of lead exposure, including exposure due to recent home renovations; and previous blood lead measurements. Particularly important is a detailed description of the condition of the child's primary residence and other places where the child spends time. All 168 hours of the week must be accounted for. Occupational histories of adults within the household and residing at other places the child visits are necessary. During the physical examination, particular attention is directed to the neurologic examination and psychosocial and language development. Neuropsychologic and neurobehavioral assessments are indicated in children with blood lead levels ≥20 µg/dL whole blood, both at the time of diagnosis and as the child approaches school age. When these assessments suggest that the child is at high risk for future learning problems, other assessments during the early school years are often necessary to facilitate an appropriate educational program. When language delay is detected, prompt referral to the appropriate program is made at the time the delay is first identified. When these problems are recognized, more formal neurocognitive evaluation should be made and subjects should be referred to an infants and toddlers program, an early intervention program, or

Head Start as appropriate. If there are nutritional problems, referral to a Women, Infants, and Children (WIC) program should be made. All cases should be reported to the appropriate health authority, which usually has the responsibility for the evaluation and enforcement of any ordinances on lead abatement. The local public health authority needs to be closely involved, because the main thrust of management is to reduce the child's exposure to environmental lead. Nutritional counseling should be conducted as described above. If the history suggests that deteriorated old house paint is not a likely source of lead, other sources (see Chapter 4) should be considered. Determination of PbB in all family members may point to a source common to all. Sometimes the index case is a pet (Marino et al., 1990).

Follow-Up

At each subsequent visit, nutritional, environmental, and behavioral (hand-to-mouth activity) data are reviewed. Progress may be gauged by the trends in paired serial blood lead and EP measurements. Certain basic information is updated to determine whether environmental exposure in the child's home has changed for the better or worse in order to ascertain whether any recent renovations have either taken place or are planned for the near future. When the address changes, a detailed history should be taken with regard to the presence and extent of scaling paint on interior and exterior surfaces. Likewise, any new secondary addresses should be identified and described. It sometimes occurs that the major source of environmental lead is at a babysitter's house and not at the primary residence; in this case, a change in babysitter is in order. One should inquire and observe during the visit whether the child's hand-to-mouth activity has increased, decreased, or remained constant in intensity. Diet should be reviewed at each visit, particularly with regard to calcium, iron, and fat intake, with particular attention to any improvements in children found initially to be iron deficient or to be receiving diets that are either deficient or grossly excessive in calcium. In those found to be iron deficient, studies in animals suggest that it may be prudent to give prophylactic amounts of copper as found in vitamin and mineral preparations together with therapeutic amounts of iron. Housecleaning techniques with regard to the frequency of cleaning and the use of high-phosphate detergents, as well as the areas cleaned (floors, woodwork, banisters, window sills and wells, etc.), are reviewed in detail at each visit. Among older children, school placement and progress in school tends to replace hand-to-mouth activity as a concern. Any change in occupation or hobbies involving potential lead exposure in an adult household member is also checked at each visit. The most important aspect of follow-up is to determine trends in blood lead and EP concentrations over time and to evaluate these in relation to changes in exposure, diet, and hand-to-mouth activity.

There probably is no single schedule for follow-up visits that is appropriate for all children. In the selection of an initial schedule, the age of the child, intensity of exposure, intensity of hand-to-mouth activity, and history of parental compliance, if known, are the important factors in determining the frequency of follow-up visits. Epidemiologic data show that blood lead concentrations increase steadily between 6 and 18 months and decline slowly, particularly after 3 years of age (Dietrich, Berger, Succop, Hammond, & Bornschein, 1993). Consequently, the younger the child, particularly toddlers less than 24 months of age, the more frequent should be the follow-up visits. The more intense the exposure and the greater the hand-to-mouth activity, the more closely the child will need to be followed. Also, children with sickle cell disease who live in old houses require particularly close follow-up because the clinical symptoms of lead poisoning and sickle cell disease may be almost indistinguishable (Nelson & Chisolm, 1986). When it is known that a family has definite plans to move, a wise precaution is to test the child a month after the move, because this may entail a change in the intensity of exposure. In general, the child might be tested at 4- to 6-week intervals during the first 3 months of follow-up in order to establish the trend in serial blood lead and EP measurements. When these measurements remain stable or decline over time, less frequent blood lead and EP tests will be needed, perhaps every 3 months during the first year of follow-up. If there is continued improvement, the intervals can be reduced to every 4 months. If the child moves from unsafe housing to safe, modern housing without lead paint hazards, and blood lead has shown a steady downward trend, such a child might need to be tested only once or twice a year to 5 or 6 years of age. As the child approaches school age, formal psychometric evaluation takes precedence over questions related to exposure in order to identify any learning handicaps that may be emerging and that may require special educational management. Additional information on screening is provided in Chapter 4.

PHARMACOLOGY OF CHELATING AGENTS

Four drugs (Table 3) are used to treat lead poisoning. None of these should be given to outpatients who are concurrently overexposed to lead. These drugs, which bind or chelate lead, deplete the soft tissues of lead and thereby reduce its acute toxicity, which is the primary goal of chelation therapy. Although these agents are effective in reducing lead concentrations in most soft tissues, their efficacy for reducing skeletal deposits, where the bulk of the body lead burden is located, is

Table 3. Chelating agents used in treating children with lead poisoning

Product name	Generic name	Chemical name	Abbreviation
Calcium disodium versenate	Edetate calcium disodium	Calcium disodium ethylenediamine-tetraacetate	CaNa$_2$EDTA
BAL in oil	Dimercaprol	2,3-Dimercapto-1-propanol	BAL
Cuprimine[a]	D-Penicillamine	3-Mercapto-D-valine	PCA
Chemet[b]	Succimer	Meso-2,3-dimercapto-succinic acid	DMSA

Adapted from CDC (1991a).
[a]Not approved by FDA for treatment of lead poisoning.
[b]Approved by the FDA for treatment of children with blood lead ≥45 μg Pb/dL whole blood.

quite limited. The rise in blood lead concentration that follows a course of chelation therapy is thought to result—in the absence of reexposure—from internal redistribution of lead from the larger skeletal deposits to the blood and other soft tissues. All drugs have potential side effects. Although a full discussion of the pharmacologic characteristics of these drugs is beyond the scope of this text, some are described below, with emphasis on precautions and potential side effects. (For a more complete discussion, see Klassen [1990]; Piomelli, Rosen, Chisolm, & Graef [1984].) In outpatients in whom chelation therapy would be inappropriate because of overexposure to lead, emphasis is placed on reducing the child's overexposure. Depending on circumstances, this may sometimes be accomplished by moving furniture in front of walls or windows where there is scaling paint. One may attempt to relocate the child temporarily to safe housing with a relative. If there is not a great deal of scaling paint, one can reduce the exposure by a thorough professional cleanup in which the house is first vacuumed thoroughly (ceilings, walls, floors, window and door units) with a high-efficiency particle accumulator (HEPA) vacuum, followed by a scrub-down with high-phosphate detergents, followed approximately 24 hours later by a second HEPA vacuuming. Such a cleanup would be the most effective way to at least temporarily reduce the child's exposure to lead. For hospitalized children, such a cleanup in the home is also advisable before they return home.

BAL

Two molecules of dimercaprol (British Anti-Lewisite, or BAL) combine with one atom of heavy metal to form a stable complex. (See Table 4.) BAL enhances both urinary and fecal excretion of lead. Because BAL is predominantly excreted in bile, it can be administered in the presence of renal impairment. BAL is available only in peanut oil for intramuscular administration; therefore, it may not be used in children who are

Table 4. Suggested dosage schedule for chelating agents in children

Chelating agent	Dosage	Administration
BAL-CaNa₂EDTA in combination Patient with PbB ≥90–100 µg/dL whole blood	BAL[a] 83 mg/m² of body surface area/dose (IM) CaNa₂EDTA[b] 250 mg/m² of body surface area/dose (IM or IV)	For the first dose, inject BAL (IM) only; beginning 4 hr later and every 4 hr thereafter for 5 days, inject BAL and CaNa₂EDTA simultaneously at separate and deep IM sites; rotate injection sites. Alternatively, CaNa₂EDTA may be administered by continuous intravenous infusion or in divided doses IV through a heparin lock; monitor electrocardiogram continuously. Second course needed only if immediate post-treatment value ≥100 µg/dL whole blood; allow 3- to 4-day interval between courses.
CaNa₂EDTA only Patient with PbB 70-90/100 µg/dL whole blood	500 mg/m² of body surface area/dose q12h (deep IM) for 5 days	IM injection simpler in young children, but if IV route preferred, as in adults, infuse each dose over a 6-hr period; may be immediately followed by oral DMSA. Second course of CaNa₂EDTA only may be used in patients not responsive to oral DMSA.
Meso-2,3-dimercaptosuccinic acid (DMSA)[c]	1050 mg/m²/day orally in three divided doses first 5 days, then reduce dose to 700 mg/m²/day orally in two divided doses for the next 14–21 days. Allow 2 weeks between courses	Available in 100-mg capsules. If child cannot take capsules, empty contents into small volume of ginger ale, fruit punch (room temperature), or puréed fruit; administer suspension PO within 5 min of mixing. Use syringe in young infants if necessary.
D-Penicillamine[d]	500 mg/m² of body surface area/day for long-term oral therapy	Give entire daily dose on empty stomach 2 hr before breakfast; contents of capsule may be mixed in a small volume of chilled puréed fruit or fruit juice immediately prior to administration. Give 25 mg pyridoxine concurrently.

Warning: Do not give chelating agents if patient is overexposed to lead (see text).

[a]BAL: The FDA recommends a dosage for adults of 2.5 mg/kg of body weight/dose every 4 hr. In "standard man" (70 kg, 1.73 m²), this is equivalent to approximately 100 mg/m² of body surface area/dose or about 20% higher than the dose recommended here for children.

[b]CaNa₂EDTA: Edathamil calcium-disodium (Versenate) is available in 20% solution. For IM use, add sufficient lidocaine to yield a final concentration of 0.5% lidocaine. IM injection is more convenient in children and permits better control of IV fluids, a vital consideration in cases of encephalopathy.

[c]DMSA: This is the preferred choice when PbB < 70 µg/dL whole blood.

[d]D-Penicillamine: Available in 125- and 250-mg capsules. It is approved by FDA for several uses but is not approved for use in lead poisoning. It has generally been used in children with PbB < 45 µg Pb/dL whole blood.

allergic to peanuts or peanut products. Some clinicians recommend that BAL be reserved for life-threatening situations in patients with glucose-6-phosphate dehydrogenase deficiency because it is suspected of causing hemolysis in such patients. Medicinal iron must never be administered during BAL treatment, because the combination of iron and BAL has been implicated in serious reactions. Edge and Somers (1948) found that iron and BAL form a complex that is more toxic than iron or BAL alone. Chisolm (1968) observed two children who inadvertently received iron during BAL-CaNa₂EDTA therapy, one by the oral route and the other by the parenteral route. In both children, vomiting intensified, metabolic evidence of lead toxicity increased, urinary excretion of lead decreased, and the rate of fall in blood lead concentration decreased. If iron deficiency coexists, it should not be treated with iron until after BAL therapy has been completed. Between 30% and 50% of patients receiving BAL will experience side effects. There may be mild febrile reactions and transient elevations of serum transaminases. Careful intravenous hydration coupled with restricted oral fluid intake can largely circumvent gastrointestinal distress (nausea and vomiting).

CaNa₂EDTA

Only CaNa₂EDTA can be used for the treatment of lead poisoning; Na₂EDTA (disodium edetate) should never be used to treat lead poisoning because it binds calcium and so can induce hypocalcemia and the associated adverse effects, such as convulsions, irregular heartbeat, and tetany (Klassen, 1990). (See Table 4.) CaNa₂EDTA increases urinary excretion 20- to 50-fold in seriously ill patients. It removes lead only from the extracellular compartment, because it does not enter cells. The preferred route of administration is intravenous. It can be given as a continuous infusion over 24 hours, or it can be given in divided doses through a heparin lock over 30–60 minutes per dose. It must never be injected rapidly. When administered intramuscularly, it must be mixed with lidocaine (or procaine) so that the final concentration of lidocaine is 0.5%. This reduces pain and may be more convenient in young, asymptomatic toddlers. The intramuscular route may be necessary in severely ill patients if there is a need to restrict fluids to an amount less than that required for dilution of CaNa₂EDTA for intravenous administration. CaNa₂EDTA should never be given orally, because it enhances absorption of lead from the gut. During therapy with CaNa₂EDTA, urine output, urine sediment, blood urea nitrogen (BUN), serum creatinine, and hepatocellular enzyme levels should be monitored prior to treatment and on the 3rd and 5th days of therapy. The appearance of protein or formed elements in the urinary sediment and rising BUN and serum creatinine reflect impending renal failure, which is the most serious toxicity associated with inappropriately excessive or prolonged administration of $CaNa_2EDTA$. $CaNa_2EDTA$ at a current dosage level of 1000 mg/m²/day for 5 days is regularly associated with a 30%–40% decrease in plasma zinc, an approximately 30% increase in serum transaminases, and an approximately 25% decrease in serum alkaline phosphatase. These changes are reversible within 3–4 days after a 5-day course of $CaNa_2EDTA$. If the patient's nutritional status is marginal, oral supplementation with prophylactic amounts of zinc (10 mg elemental zinc, tid) and copper (2 mg elemental copper) given as acetates with meals may be helpful.

D-Penicillamine

The U.S. Food and Drug Administration (FDA) has approved *D*-penicillamine for the treatment of Wilson's disease, cystinuria, and severe active rheumatoid arthritis, but not for the treatment of lead poisoning. (See Table 4.) This drug can be and has been given orally for periods of weeks up to 3–6 months and has generally been used in children with blood lead levels <45 µg/dL whole blood. It enhances urinary excretion of lead, although not as effectively as $CaNa_2EDTA$. It is not specific for lead and is associated with modest increases in the urinary excretion of copper and zinc. It is administered orally, with the usual dose being 500 mg/m²/day, given in divided dose for 4–12 weeks. Side effects occur in as many as 33% of patients given the drug (Shannon, Graef, & Lovejoy, 1988). The main side effects are reactions resembling those of penicillin sensitivity and include rashes, leukopenia, thrombocytopenia, hematuria, proteinuria, and hepatocellular enzyme elevations. Of greatest concern, however, are isolated reports of Stevens–Johnson syndrome and nephrotoxicity, possibly due to hypersensitivity. For these reasons, patients must be carefully monitored for clinically obvious side effects, and frequent blood counts and urinalyses should be performed. During the first month of therapy, monitoring should be conducted on a weekly basis and on a monthly basis thereafter. The drug should not be given on an outpatient basis where exposure to lead is continuing and should not be administered to patients with known sensitivity to penicillin.

DMSA

Meso-2,3-dimercaptosuccinic acid (DMSA, also called succimer), a water-soluble analog of BAL, is an effective oral chelating agent for lead. Its selectivity for lead is high, whereas its ability to chelate essential trace metals in children is low. Although studies on the efficacy of succimer are limited, it appears to be quite promising. It has a much higher therapeutic index than BAL and is absorbed from the gastrointestinal tract (Aposhian & Aposhian, 1990). There is some preliminary evidence that suggests, but does not conclusively demonstrate, that administration of DMSA concurrently with the administration of lead to human adult volunteers may be associated with increased absorption and retention of lead (Smith, Markowitz, Crick, Rosen, & Flegal, 1994). Further study on this important issue is needed; meanwhile, it would be prudent to administer this drug to outpatients only if overexposure to lead can be precluded. To date, no serious adverse reactions have been reported. Most of the reactions that have been reported, including those related to gastrointestinal distress, have been reported in adults. In children, extraordinary, reversible elevations in serum alkaline phosphatase have been observed. It is not clear whether this is directly related to the drug, because there is an asymptomatic entity in young children known as benign transient hyperphosphatasemia (Crofton, 1988). DMSA is administered orally and is available only in 100-mg capsules. It is preferable to calculate the dosage in children on the basis of surface area and not on the basis of body weight, which may provide insufficient dosage. In some children, two or more courses may be necessary. Dosage and schedules may be modified as more experience is gained; DMSA was approved by the FDA for the treatment of lead poisoning only in 1991. For young children who cannot swallow the capsules, DMSA can be administered by separating the capsules and suspending the medicated beads in room temperature fruit juice or ginger ale or by sprinkling them on puréed fruit. This mixing should occur within 5 minutes of administration because the drug rapidly loses its potency once removed from the capsule. Because clinical experience is limited, the full spectrum and incidence of serious adverse reactions, including the possibility of hypersensitivity or idiosyncratic reactions, have not been determined. Currently, this drug is approved for children with blood lead levels ≥45 µg/dL whole blood; however, a number of clinicians institute treatment at 40 µg/dL whole blood or lower. The upper limit of blood lead concentration at which the approved dosage is still efficacious is not known; however, reports in the clinical literature have almost exclusively involved patients (children and adults) with blood lead concentrations <100 µg/dL.

TREATMENT GUIDELINES

The most important principle in managing childhood lead poisoning is to reduce the child's exposure to environmental lead. Children with symptomatic lead poisoning should be admitted to a hospital with a pediatric intensive care unit and should receive chelation therapy. Asymptomatic children with blood lead levels ≥40–45 µg/dL whole blood are appropriate candidates for chelation therapy, but the drug must not be given to outpatients unless the child is residing in lead-safe housing as determined by professional inspection. Detailed discussion of treatment is beyond the scope of this chapter but may be found elsewhere (Chisolm & Lombeck, 1993; Mortenson & Walsen, 1993; Piomelli et al., 1984). Suggested dosage schedules are shown in Table 4.

Symptomatic Children and Asymptomatic Children with Blood Lead Concentrations ≥90–100 µg/dL Whole Blood

Because the clinical course of lead poisoning is unpredictable when blood lead concentration exceeds 90–100 µg/dL whole blood, all children should be considered as potential cases of encephalopathy and treated with combined BAL and CaNa$_2$EDTA. In this regimen, BAL is injected first and simultaneous administration of BAL and CaNa$_2$EDTA is begun 4 hours later. This is done because BAL has been shown to regenerate the sulfhydryl enzymes inhibited by lead, whereas CaNa$_2$EDTA does not. Also, this allows sufficient time to reinstitute urinary flow, which is essential before starting CaNa$_2$EDTA because CaNa$_2$EDTA is not metabolized and its elimination depends exclusively on the renal route. Because the child's neurologic and renal status, as well as fluid balance, must be carefully monitored, such children should be treated in a pediatric intensive care unit for the first 48–72 hours DMSA has not been used in symptomatic children, but has been reported to alleviate symptoms in adults. The decision to use this combination at blood lead concentrations of 70–100 µg/dL involves a choice between removal of more lead than could be achieved with CaNa$_2$EDTA alone and the pain associated with the injection of BAL. CaNa$_2$EDTA in this range has not been reported to provoke the onset of symptomatic lead poisoning; thus, it does not carry the risk of a life-threatening event. Furthermore, the adequacy of the present recommended dosage of succimer at higher blood lead concentrations has not been established. Children with acute encephalopathy often have impaired renal function. Usually, their therapy can be managed with an initial 5-day course of BAL-CaNa$_2$EDTA, followed by a 5-day course of CaNa$_2$EDTA alone (if blood lead < 100 µg/dL whole blood), and thereafter with at least one course of oral DMSA. Renal and hepatic function and serum electrolyte levels should be monitored daily during treatment with BAL-CaNa$_2$EDTA. When BAL is stopped after 2–3 days, blood lead concentration will increase, despite the fact that CaNa$_2$EDTA administration continues for the full 5 days.

Asymptomatic Children with
Blood Lead Concentrations 70–100 µg/dL Whole Blood

Experience is limited, but a few children with initial blood lead concentrations in this range have shown only a limited response to DMSA as measured by the decrease in blood lead concentration. The reasons for this are not clear. Therefore, it may be prudent to give such children an initial 5-day course of CaNa$_2$EDTA followed by a 19- to 26-day course of oral DMSA. In such children, blood lead concentration often rebounds even after this regimen to >40 µg/dL whole blood after an interval of 2–4 weeks. In such cases, a second course of oral DMSA is appropriate. When DMSA is given, complete blood counts and serum chemistries (alanine aminotransferase, aspartate aminotransferase, alkaline phosphatase) should be monitored on a weekly basis. CaNa$_2$EDTA should not be given for more than 5 successive days at the dosage shown in Table 4.

Asymptomatic Children with Blood Lead
Concentrations 40/45–69 µg/dL Whole Blood

In these children, initial experience indicates that treatment with oral DMSA is preferred. Only if the patient responds poorly should CaNa$_2$EDTA be considered in this group. The dosage and blood lead ranges shown in Table 4 represent a suggested therapeutic approach. It is known, however, that some clinicians treat children whose blood lead concentrations are lower than 40–45 µg/dL whole blood with DMSA and, in the past, with D-penicillamine, although currently DMSA may be replacing D-penicillamine in this latter group of patients.

Asymptomatic Children with Blood Lead
Concentrations 20–40/45 µg/dL Whole Blood

In this group, major emphasis is placed on modifying the child's environment, either through abatement of lead paint hazards in the child's house or through relocation to lead-safe housing. Whether treatment with DMSA offers any additional advantage to that gained by reducing the child's exposure is unknown and is currently the subject of clinical trial (NIEHS News, 1993).

Inpatient Versus Outpatient Management

Where drugs must be given by injection, as in the case of BAL and CaNa$_2$EDTA, the patient should be treated as an inpatient. In addition, symptomatic patients may require additional supportive measures. When chelation therapy is given to asymptomatic patients, therapy should be administered in lead poisoning treatment centers that are outside of the hospital. These can be found in several large urban centers. Only if the child can reside in a lead-safe residence while receiving the chelating agent should outpatient therapy be considered. Furthermore, parental compliance is necessary. It may be possible to relocate the child temporarily during chelation therapy with a relative who does live in lead-safe housing. During this interval, every effort should be made to assist the parent(s) in relocating to lead-safe housing. If renovations are made to render the primary address lead-safe, children and pregnant women should stay out of the house until both renovations and proper cleanup with high-phosphate washes and HEPA vacuum have been completed. Administration of chelation therapy will not lead to long-lasting improvement unless the child's exposure to lead is reduced.

Follow-Up of Patients Who Have Received Chelation Therapy

At the end of each treatment cycle, the blood lead concentration usually declines after $CaNa_2EDTA$ to 55%–60% of the pretreatment value and at the end of treatment with DMSA to 25%–50% of the pretreatment value. However, reequilibriation among body compartments takes place and generally results after 2–4 weeks in a rebound in blood lead concentration to approximately 70% of the pretreatment value. Blood lead levels should be checked 14 and 28 days after treatment to determine whether further treatment is indicated. Children who undergo chelation therapy require long-term follow-up. Ideally, children should never be discharged from the hospital until they can go to a lead-safe environment. Unfortunately, an emphasis on reducing the costs of medical care makes this impossible in many cases. Even so, intense effort should be made to find lead-safe housing with friends or relatives or in designated transitional housing where the child can stay until relocation is possible or until the entire abatement and postabatement cleanup process has been completed in the primary residence. The medical social service worker can be indispensable in helping the family arrange for lead-safe housing.

The child should be rechecked 2 and 4 weeks following discharge and at monthly intervals until 3 months following discharge. During this period, measurements of blood lead and EP at each visit are of great value in helping to determine whether there is internal redistribution or renewed excessive assimilation of lead. The blood lead concentration can be expected to stabilize about 4 weeks after therapy and then decline slowly if the child is only experiencing internal redistribution of lead. If this is the case, a progressive decrease in EP should accompany this rebound phenomenon. If, however, both blood lead and EP increase in comparison with the immediate post-treatment values, continuing excessive ingestion of environmental lead is strongly implicated. It is clearly implicated if the blood lead concentration increases to a value greater than the pretreatment value. Once it has been established that further chelation therapy is no longer indicated in the immediate future, the child should be followed in the same manner as that described above for children with blood lead concentrations ≥20 µg/dL whole blood who are not receiving chelation therapy.

CONCLUSIONS

The most important component of medical management is to facilitate reduction in the child's exposure to the environmental lead. In this sense, administration of chelation therapy may be considered adjunctive. Chelation therapy, when promptly administered, can be life saving and can reduce the period of morbidity. Such cases were rather common until the mid-1960s, but since the early 1990s acutely symptomatic cases have rarely been encountered in the United States, although they continue to be reported from the Third World. The rationale for administering chelation therapy to asymptomatic patients in conjunction with prompt reduction in exposure to lead is that it may reduce the period of overexposure of the brain to lead, thereby reducing the occurrence and/or severity of residua such as learning disabilities, which become evident only later, during school age. However, this has not been proven. A randomized, double-blind, placebo-controlled clinical trial is now in progress to determine whether chelation therapy with DMSA in children with blood lead concentrations of 20–44 µg/dL whole blood during the toddler stage offers any benefit in addition to that which can be obtained by reduction of exposure, which will be carried out in both the placebo and treatment groups. The benefit (if any) of DMSA will be determined by comparing neurobehavioral outcomes in the treatment and placebo groups determined at approximately 5 years of age. Some, but by no means all, states do have funding programs to facilitate abatement of lead paint hazards in old housing and/or relocation of lead-poisoned children to lead-safe housing. Clinicians must work in close concert with medical social service workers to carry this out in individual cases. For over 25 years, the American Academy of Pediatrics at both the national and state chapter levels has worked to promote screening, reporting, and hazard reduction activities for the benefit of children as a group. Pediatricians can work through their chapters to facilitate legislation where needed and to act as advocates for this and other aspects of improvements in child health. In dealing with individual children, disabilities such as learning disabilities and expressive language delay should be identified as soon as possible so that appropriate referrals can be made to infants and toddlers, early intervention, Head Start, and similar programs in the hope that such stimulation will counteract at least in part any deficits attributable to lead. Until the old, deteriorated housing in which lead toxicity occurs in the United States is rehabilitated or replaced, health care providers will continue to be faced with this problem. The data from the Third National Health and Nutrition Examination Survey (NHANES III) are encouraging (Pirkle et al., 1994). The importance of the "risk accumulator factor"—namely, the fact that one old, deteriorated house, if not properly maintained, can poison many children—must be recognized so that greater emphasis will be placed on reducing exposure rather than attempting to treat children after injury has occurred.

REFERENCES

Aposhian, H.V., & Aposhian, M.M. (1990). Meso-2,3-dimercaptosuccinic acid: Chemical, pharmacological and toxicological properties of an orally effective metal chelating agent. *Annual Reviews of Pharmacology and Toxicology, 30*, 279–306.

Bellinger, D.C., Stiles, K.M., & Needleman, H.L. (1992). Low-level lead exposure, intelligence and academic achievement: A long-term follow-up study. *Pediatrics, 90*, 855–861.

Bornschein, R.L., Succop, P.A., Kraft, K.M., Clark, C.S., Peace, B., & Hammond, P.B. (1986). Exterior surface dust lead, interior house dust lead and childhood lead exposure in an urban environment. In D.D. Hemphill (Ed.), *Trace substances in environmental health. XX. Proceedings of the University of Missouri's 20th Annual Conference* (pp. 322–332). Columbia: University of Missouri.

Centers for Disease Control and Prevention (CDC). (1991a). *Preventing lead poisoning in young children: A statement by the Centers for Disease Control.* Atlanta: U.S. Department of Health and Human Services, Public Health Service.

Centers for Disease Control and Prevention (CDC). (1991b). *Strategic plan for the elimination of childhood lead poisoning: Developed for the Risk Management Subcommittee, Committee to Coordinate Environmental Health and Related Programs.* Atlanta: U.S. Department of Health and Human Services, Public Health Service.

Chisolm, J.J., Jr. (1968). The use of chelating agents in the treatment of acute and chronic lead intoxication in childhood. *Journal of Pediatrics, 73*, 1–38.

Chisolm, J.J., Jr. (1982). Management of increased lead absorption—Illustrative cases. In J.J. Chisolm, Jr. & D.M. O'Hara (Eds.), *Lead absorption in children: Management, clinical and environmental aspects* (pp. 171–188). Baltimore: Urban & Schwarzenberg.

Chisolm, J.J., Jr., & Lombeck, I. (1993). Lead poisoning. In H.F. Eichenwald & J. Stroder (Eds.), *Pediatric therapy* (3rd ed.) (pp. 1167–1174). St. Louis, MO: C.V. Mosby.

Crofton, P.M. (1988). What is the cause of benign transient hyperphosphatasemia? A study of 35 cases. *Clinical Chemistry, 34*, 335–340.

Davies, D.J.A., Thornton, I., Watt, J.M., Culbard, E.B., Harvey, P.G., Delves, H.T., Sherlock, J.C., Smart, G.A., Thomas, J.F.A., & Quinn, M.J. (1990). Lead intake and blood lead in two-year-old U.K. urban children. *Science of the Total Environment, 90*, 13–29.

Dietrich, K.N., Berger, O.G., Succop, P.A., Hammond, P.B., & Bornschein, R.L. (1993). The developmental consequences of low to moderate prenatal and postnatal lead exposure: Intellectual attainment on the Cincinnati Lead Study Cohort following school entry. *Neurotoxicology and Teratology, 17*, 37–44.

Edge, M.D., & Somers, G.F. (1948). The effect of dimercaprol (BAL) in acute iron poisoning. *Quarterly Journal of Pharmacology, 21*, 364.

Goldstein, G.W. (1992). Developmental neurobiology of lead toxicity. In H.L. Needleman (Ed.), *Human lead exposure* (pp. 125–136). Boca Raton, FL: CRC Press.

Hastka, J., Lasserre, J-J., Schwarzbeck, A., & Hehlmann, R. (1994). Central role of zinc protoporphyrin in staging iron deficiency. *Clinical Chemistry, 40*, 768–773.

Klander, D.S., & Petering, H.G. (1977). Anemia of lead intoxication: A role for copper. *Journal of Nutrition, 107*, 1779–1785.

Klassen, C.D. (1990). Heavy metals and heavy-metal antagonists. In A.G. Gilman, T.W. Rall, A.S. Nies, & P. Taylor (Eds.), *The pharmacological basis of therapeutics* (8th ed.) (pp. 1592–1614). New York: Pergamon Press.

Mahaffey, K.R. (1981). Nutritional factors and lead poisoning. *Nutrition Reviews, 39*, 353–361.

Marino, P.E., Landrigan, P.J., Graef, J., Nussbaum, A., Bayan, G., Boch, K., & Boch, S. (1990). A case report of lead paint poisoning during renovation of a victorian farmhouse. *American Journal of Public Health, 80*, 1183–1185.

Markowitz, M.E., Bijur, P.E., Ruff, H., & Rosen, J.F. (1993). Effects of calcium disodium versenate ($CaNa_2EDTA$) chelation in moderate childhood lead poisoning. *Pediatrics, 92*, 265–271.

Mortenson, M.E., & Walson, P.D. (1993). Chelation therapy for childhood lead poisoning. *Clinical Pediatrics, 5*, 284–291.

Nelson, M.S., & Chisolm, J.J., Jr. (1986). Lead toxicity masquerading as sickle cell crisis. *Annals of Emergency Medicine, 15*(6), 748–750.

NIEHS News. (1993). Succimer gets TLC. *Environmental Health Perspectives, 101*, 284–285.

Oski, F. (1993). Iron deficiency in infancy and childhood. *New England Journal of Medicine, 329*, 190–193.

Piomelli, S., Rosen, J.F., Chisolm, J.J., Jr., & Graef, J.W. (1984). Management of childhood lead poisoning. *Journal of Pediatrics, 105*, 523–532.

Pirkle, J.L., Brody, D.J., Gunter, E.W., Kramer, R.A., Paschal, D.C., Flegal, K.M., & Matte, T.D. (1994). The decline in blood lead levels in the United States: The National Health and Nutrition Examination Surveys (NHANES). *Journal of the American Medical Association, 272*, 284–291.

Rabinowitz, M.B., Wetherill, G.W., & Kopple, J.D. (1976). Kinetic analysis of lead metabolism in healthy humans. *Journal of Clinical Investigation, 58*, 260–270.

Shannon, N., Graef, J., & Lovejoy, F.H., Jr. (1988). Efficacy and toxicity of D-penicillamine in low-level lead poisoning. *Journal of Pediatrics, 112*, 799–804.

Smith, D.R., Markowitz, M.E., Crick, J., Rosen, J.F., & Flegal, A.R. (1994). The effects of succimer on the absorption of lead in adults determined by using the stable isotope ^{204}Pb. *Environmental Research, 67*, 39–53.

Todd, C.A., & Chettle, D.R. (1994). In vivo X-ray fluorescence of lead in bone: Review and current issues. *Environmental Health Perspectives, 102,* 172–177.

Ziegler, E.E., Edwards, B.B., Jensen, R.L., Mahaffey, K.R., & Fomon, S.J. (1978). Absorption and retention of lead by infants. *Pediatric Research, 12,* 29–34.

9

ENVIRONMENTAL ABATEMENT

James G. Linakis
Angela C. Anderson
Siegfried M. Pueschel

L ead poisoning in childhood is presently known to result from exposure to lead from one or more of a number of sources: lead-based paint, lead-containing dust, lead-contaminated soil or water, and lead-polluted air (Rabinowitz, Leviton, Needleman, Bellinger, & Waternaux, 1985). As has been pointed out elsewhere in this volume, the problem of atmospheric lead has been largely reduced through the elimination of lead from gasoline. Coinciding with that elimination, there has been a dramatic reduction in blood lead levels during the same period (Annest, 1983). Presently, exposure to lead from paint (including that in dust and soil) and water represents the major cause of lead poisoning in children. Paint in particular is an exceptionally troublesome source (Schwartz & Levin, 1991). Indeed, it is thought that nearly 52% of occupied residential units in the United States, or 42 million dwellings, contain lead-based paint. Nearly 6 million children under the age of 7 years are thought to live in those houses containing the highest lead content (Agency for Toxic Substances and Disease Registry, 1988), and there is strong evidence suggesting that 3 million children in the United States have blood lead levels greater than the currently accepted lower level of concern (10 µg/dL) (Goodman, Shultz, Klitzman, Kimmelblatt, & Spadaro, 1993).

There has been a significant amount of discussion regarding the optimum means for diminishing the environmental lead to which children are exposed. Fundamentally, the debate has centered around the desirability of completely removing all lead sources to which children might be exposed versus the practicality of erecting barriers that would prevent children from reaching the sources of lead, with consideration of several intermediate measures. As mentioned above, the area in which the most improvement in lead exposure reduction has been noted in the United States has been that of atmospheric lead contamination. It had long been recognized that lead-containing gasoline represented the major source of lead in ambient air, and although attempts to alleviate the problem were aided by intermediate steps, such as catalytic converters in automobiles (which were not specifically intended to reduce lead pollution), the nearly complete elimination of lead from most gasoline was the step to which was attributed the dramatic decrease of average blood lead concentrations (Annest, 1983; Davis, Elias, & Grant, 1993). Unfortunately, the problems associated with abatement of lead from water, soil, dust, and existing paint coatings are enormously complex and expensive to overcome.

The present chapter discusses abatement of lead hazards from each of the major sources of lead exposure. Although much remains to be learned about the most effective means of abatement and there will undoubtedly continue to be plentiful debate regarding the appropriate roles of complete abatement versus cost-effective abatement, this chapter describes a practical and effective set of possibilities for the management of environmental abatement.

ENVIRONMENTAL INSPECTION

Paint

In its 1991 statement on the prevention of lead poisoning in children, the U.S. Centers for Disease Control and Prevention (CDC) recommended environmental intervention for children with blood lead levels of ≥ 20 µg/dL, or of ≥ 15 µg/dL that persist, but recognized that limited resources may shift this intervention level higher in many communities (CDC, 1991). Environmental investigation should begin concomitantly with parental education regarding the causes and effects of lead poisoning, the likely course of treatment and follow-up, the role of nutrition in decreasing lead poisoning, and resources to which parents can turn for assistance in dealing with the complex issues of lead poisoning and lead abatement. Typically, in the case of the lead-poisoned child, inspection is carried out by public health officials (see Chapter 11), although commercial inspections are available. The goal of environmental inspection is to ascertain the most likely sources of exposure to lead, particularly high-dose exposure. This involves investigation of the child's home and other environments in which the child spends a significant amount of time. Inspection should include both the interior and the exterior of the structure(s) in question and should evaluate dust, soil, and water as well as painted surfaces.

In inspecting painted surfaces, all surfaces are initially assumed to contain lead unless constructed after 1977, the year in which the addition of lead to house paint was definitively prohibited. Inspections are best performed on representative surfaces, and special attention should be paid to those surfaces most easily mouthed by a child, such as railings, banisters, and window sills. A comprehensive inspection will consist of testing the following surfaces in each room of the dwelling: walls, ceilings, sills, wells, sashes, railings (interior and exterior), stairs, banisters, floors, doors and door jambs, door casings, and woodwork and molding. On the exterior, walls, doors and door frames, window frames, and trim should all be inspected. In addition, other suspect painted objects may require testing, including cribs and toys.

There are several methods available for determining the lead content of paint. *X-ray fluorescence* (XRF) permits analysis of intact paint using a handheld device. The test uses a radioactive source (usually cobalt-57) that excites lead atoms in the target sample. As the atoms return to their normal state, they emit X rays that are characteristic of lead. The instrument measures these X rays and gives a reading that indicates the lead concentration in mg/cm^2. For most XRF devices, 10 mg/cm^2 is the maximum reading registered by the device, although actual concentrations may be considerably higher. Because of its convenience, XRF is commonly used to inspect for lead. The direct reading devices have a relatively wide margin of error (especially at lower levels of lead). However, the spectrum analyzer, although more accurate, is considerably more expensive. XRF devices are intended for use only by trained personnel, and when used properly offer rapid testing with a reasonable degree of accuracy. The 1985 CDC statement on lead recommended a value of 0.7 mg/cm^2 as the maximum level of lead in paint in a residence by XRF (CDC, 1985), although the U.S. Department of Housing and Urban Development (HUD) standard, as mandated by Congress, is 1.0 mg/cm^2 (Davis et al., 1993; U.S. Department of Housing and Urban Development, 1990a, 1990b). A number of states have enacted their own XRF standard, ranging from 0.7 to 1.2 mg/cm^2.

Atomic absorption spectrometry permits more precise quantitation of lead in paint. It generally must be used if an XRF device is not available or produces ambiguous results. During this test, a paint sample is digested in acid, then atomized in the flame of a burner. Atoms that consequently reach an excited state are measured by a detector in the device. This method requires that a paint chip sample be collected from each representative area to be analyzed. Each paint chip should be removed in such a manner as to ensure that the sample contains all layers of paint. Although the atomic absorption method permits more accurate quantitative analysis, it requires highly specialized laboratory equipment and personnel and is both expensive and time consuming. The HUD guidelines use a standard of 0.5% lead by weight for this method of analysis.

As with XRF, chemical *spot tests* can be performed on site. However, they permit a qualitative assessment only for the presence or absence of lead and are somewhat subjective in their interpretation. Performance of the test involves placement of a chemical (generally sodium rhodizonate) on either intact paint, nonintact paint, or a scratch made through intact paint. If the chemical turns a certain color (red in the case of sodium rhodizonate), the presence of lead is confirmed. In many regions, negative or ambiguous results are confirmed with XRF or laboratory analysis.

Dust and Soil

It is now recognized that a significant number of children with lead poisoning are poisoned by lead-contaminated dust ingested through normal childhood hand-to-mouth activity. On occasion, this dust comes from lead-contaminated soil that is tracked into the house or from the clothes of a parent who works in a lead-related industry. Consequently, the distinction between soil and dust as exposure sources may not be as clear as initially thought. Industrial and mobile sources have contributed to soil lead levels in some regions. More commonly, however, the source of lead in both soil and dust has been identified to be lead-based paint (CDC, 1991). The normal aging process of both interior and exterior paint causes flaking and chalking, which may produce lead dust inside a residence and can contaminate soil adjacent to exterior painted walls. The U.S. Environmental Protection Agency (EPA) has provided some technical support to HUD regarding lead-based paint abatement, but its main focus on soil lead has been with regard to Superfund sites. For these sites, the EPA Office of Solid Waste and Emergency Response specified 1,000 ppm as a trigger concentration for effecting cleanup efforts and 500 ppm as the remediation goal (U.S. EPA, 1989/1990). The EPA has subsequently published guidelines for the management of soil lead hazards (Title X, Housing and Community Development Act of 1992, PL 102-550: Section H03 Guidelines). According to these guidelines, soil lead concentrations < 400 ppm do not require intervention, whereas concentrations of 400–5,000 ppm require remediation in those areas frequented by children. It is important to note that these levels are intended as guidelines and not as binding or enforceable standards. Although many municipalities use these standards, others have adopted separate criteria.

Interior Dust   Testing for lead in interior dust is generally performed by obtaining a sample with either the wipe method using a premoistened towelette or the vacuum method (Que Hee et al., 1985). Unfortunately, there are few standards for these two methods of dust collection, and a 1994 study concluded that a commonly used vacuum method may underestimate lead loadings when compared to a frequently used wipe-sampling method (Farfel et al., 1994). Again, samples are collected from the highest risk areas, including floors, window sills and wells, and carpets and upholstered furniture, if present. Areas of focus should include the child's bedroom and any rooms used frequently for play. Large pieces of material are removed from the sample, and the samples are analyzed for lead content with XRF or atomic absorption spectrometry.

Soil and Exterior Dust   The lead content of soil is most frequently determined with XRF, although laboratory methods such as atomic absorption are also used. Soil samples are collected from each side of the structure and from areas of the yard used for play. Exterior dust samples are collected by vacuuming or wet-wiping.

Drinking Water

Although lead in drinking water is not the predominant source of lead for most lead-poisoned children, the EPA has estimated that between 20% and 40% of the average blood lead level in U.S. children is the result of lead in their drinking water (U.S. EPA, 1990). Source water—groundwater and water in reservoirs—rarely contains high levels of lead. In fact, lead in drinking water is generally secondary to the contamination of water by lead-containing components of the plumbing system. The chemical reaction of water with lead-containing pipes, lead connectors, and other lead-containing plumbing components, such as solder and brass, permits the entry of variable amounts of lead into drinking water. Consequently, it has been demonstrated that the concentration of lead in drinking water varies from one municipality to another and even from one residence within a given municipality to another, depending on such factors as age and condition of the plumbing, pH and temperature of the water, and the amount of time water stands in the contaminated plumbing (Davis et al., 1993).

To determine the highest levels of lead exposure in a dwelling's drinking water, a water sample is taken from the tap or taps after water has remained static in the pipes for several (at least 6) hours overnight. A second sample, obtained after the water has been allowed to flow freely for 3–5 minutes, demonstrates if flushing the line decreases lead content significantly. Lead in drinking water is most frequently quantitated using atomic absorption spectrometry.

In 1975, the EPA established the national primary drinking water regulation for lead at 50 µg/L (U.S. EPA, 1975). Subsequently, in 1986, a ban on the use of lead pipes and lead solder in plumbing that comes into contact with drinking water was issued (Safe Drinking Water Act Amendments, 1986), and in 1991 the national primary drinking water regulation was revised downward to an action level of ≥15 µg/L at the 90th percentile of sampled taps (U.S. EPA, 1991). This level is enforceable, but is primarily meant to direct the treatment practices of public water suppliers in reducing the corrosivity of water and consequently the amount of lead that leaches into the drinking water (Davis et al., 1993).

ENVIRONMENTAL ABATEMENT

Paint

Historically, several approaches to the abatement of lead-based paint have been taken. Even today there is widespread disagreement among industrial engineers, clinical toxicologists, and public health officials regarding the optimum means for remediation of the lead-based paint problem. Not only do experts disagree on the means by which lead-based paint should be removed, but they disagree on the extent to which it should be removed. However, there does seem to be general agreement that new techniques must be developed to allow for the rapid, safe, economical, and environmentally sound alleviation of the problem.

To a large extent, the realization of the need for new abatement methods came about as a result of a study of children in Baltimore who had pretreatment blood lead concentrations of ≥50 µg/dL. Of the children studied, 154 were discharged to old housing that had reportedly undergone lead paint abatement. Among those children, blood lead levels of ≥50 µg/dL recurred 127 times in 75 children; in contrast, among the 20 children discharged to housing that never contained lead-based paint, there were no such recurrences and blood lead concentrations were significantly lower (Chisolm, 1986; Chisolm, Mellits, & Quaskey, 1985).

Before discussing specific means of lead-based paint abatement, it is important to note the distinction between a lead-safe environment and one that is lead-free. According to public health officials in many communities, acceptable abatement consists of rendering housing lead safe. *Lead-safe* describes a dwelling that has undergone sufficient lead hazard reduction to ensure that no significant environmental lead hazard is present. This includes scraping of peeling lead-based paint and covering of the remainder with fresh paint or encapsulants such as wallpaper or wood paneling. *Lead-free*, however, refers to a dwelling that either contains no lead or contains lead in amounts less than the maximum acceptable environmental level established by local or federal authorities. Obviously, rendering an older home lead-free can be an extremely time consuming and expensive process. Nevertheless, once such complete abatement is carried out, there is no future risk to the children living in the house or to the generations of children who may live in the house in the future. Unfortunately, the economic issue is a real one, as discussed in Chapter 12, and complete abatement of all lead-containing paint may not be a practical short-term goal.

As mentioned above, in the past, numerous methodologies have been attempted to abate lead-based paint. It is now widely recognized that several of these methods pose a danger to both the person undertaking the abatement process and others in the vicinity. These unacceptable methods of lead-based paint abatement include the following:

1. The use of open-flame torches to burn off paint, because this process produces high lead concentrations in the air
2. Sanding or grinding paint without the use of an industrial high-efficiency particle air filter (HEPA) vacuum (see below), because this results in a high concentration of lead dust particles that spread throughout the vicinity (Grondona, 1993; Zedd, Walker, Hernandez, & Thomas, 1993)
3. Uncontained waterblasting, sandblasting, or dry-scraping without concomitant misting, because this also produces high concentrations of lead that can contaminate nearby buildings, streets, and yards

Repainting over lead-based paint or covering with wallpaper or contact paper should be viewed as only a short-term measure to reduce the immediate risk of lead dust, because the underlying lead-based paint continues to chalk and contaminate the environment (Keck, 1990).

Actions that constitute acceptable modalities of lead-based paint abatement vary from one locale to another. However, three specific techniques—replacement, encapsulation, and paint removal—have the widest degree of acceptance.

1. *Replacement* of old surfaces previously painted with lead-based paint such as windows, doors, and trim, though effective in definitively removing lead, is extremely expensive and time consuming. Furthermore, whereas replacement of the aforementioned items is

at times practical, replacement of ceilings and walls, which may also contain high concentrations of lead, often is infeasible.

2. *Encapsulation*, at the present time, can rarely be viewed as a permanent solution. However, when surfaces are encapsulated to the extent that children are denied access to the surface's lead-based paint and dust is sealed and made inaccessible, the resultant degree of safety can be considerable as well as long term. Encapsulants are classified as rigid (e.g., paneling, sheet rock) and flexible (e.g., fiberglass sheets that are mounted on specialized materials and coated with additional material). Although encapsulation was previously disparaged because of the ineffectiveness of early attempts to contain dust, new methods of encapsulation are currently being developed that may offer an effective and cost-efficient solution to the lead-based paint problem. It should be noted, however, that simple spot scraping and painting over of peeling lead-based paint is an entirely inadequate means of abatement and should not be included among the encapsulation methods.

3. *Paint removal* may be performed by one of several methods as discussed below. Although frequently time consuming and labor intensive, paint removal is one of the few ways to ensure that lead-based paint does not continue to be a threat to future generations of children living in the housing unit. Virtually all methods of paint removal require workers to be meticulous in their labor and painstaking in postabatement cleanup.

When to Abate   In its 1991 statement, the CDC recommended environmental intervention when children living in the environment are discovered to have lead levels of ≥20 µg/dL, or when their levels are ≥15 µg/dL and persist at that level (CDC, 1991). As a matter of practicality, however, the statement was intended to acknowledge that, in many municipalities, resources are limited with regard to both inspection of dwellings and abatement operations. Consequently, the recommendation was made that when resources are limited, they should be focused on those children with the highest blood lead concentrations. Although seemingly practical, this suggestion risks interpretation, which may permit long-term inactivity with regard to definitive abatement in these cases, thus permitting the persistence of lead in the household. Unfortunately, the issue of financing inspection and abatement is a complex one (see Chapter 12) and one that is managed in diverse ways in different locales.

Abatement Procedures   When a child is recognized to have lead poisoning, particularly when the blood lead concentration is ≥20 µg/dL, the first phase of management should be removal of the child from the lead-containing environment or removal of the lead from the child's environment. Because in many regions the scarcity of lead-safe housing precludes relocating all children with lead poisoning from their dwellings, often emergency abatement measures must be taken to temporarily attenuate the lead hazard. These include immediate, careful removal of paint chips and dust abatement through wet-mopping of floors and wet-wiping of window sills and wells with high-phosphate cleaners. In addition, toys and baby bottles, pacifiers, and other frequently mouthed objects should be washed thoroughly on a daily basis, and children's hands should be washed frequently (particularly before meals). Inside play areas should be restricted to locations without peeling or chipping paint and outside play should be confined to areas away from those immediately adjacent to the dwelling.

These measures should by no means be considered to be a definitive solution to lead-based paint contamination of a dwelling. On the contrary, permanent abatement is considered to have occurred only when all lead-based paint is entirely removed or made permanently inaccessible. As mentioned above, disagreement exists regarding the necessity for permanent abatement when lead poisoning is marked by relatively low blood lead concentrations, but permanent abatement is the only way to ensure the safety of the dwelling for future occupants.

Several acceptable methods of lead-based paint removal have been used, although these vary from region to region and even between lead abatement contractors in a given area. Regardless of the technique used, proper abatement includes a number of specific steps as discussed in the 1991 CDC statement.

First, abatement of lead-based paint should be carried out only by workers who are trained, skilled, and experienced in abatement procedures. In many states, it is required that such workers be licensed or certified by the state. Workers should be familiar with the health effects of lead and proficient in the conduct of worker protection procedures (including respirator use), containment operations, and hazardous waste disposal.

Second, abatement proceedings should be conducted only after painstaking efforts have been taken to *ensure that occupants are not present during lead hazard reduction* (Amitai, Brown, Graef, & Cosgrove, 1991). In addition, there should be meticulous protection of abatement workers and their families from the lead dust that is generated during abatement. The latter can be carried out by ensuring that workers in the abatement area be attired in disposable coveralls, shoe coverings, hair coverings, gloves, goggles, and a properly fitted, negative pressure, half-face respirator with HEPA filter cartridges. Full-face, negative pressure, and supplied-air respirators are also acceptable, although they are considerably less popular because of their inconvenience. Prior to beginning work, workers should change into clean work clothing and don their respirators before entering the work area. Upon leaving the work area, workers should HEPA-vacuum heavily contaminated protective work garments and then remove protective clothing and gear in the "dirty" area of a designated changing area. Workers should not be permitted to eat, drink, or smoke in the work area, because the hazard of lead dust ingestion is great. After leaving the work area and removing protective gear, workers should at the very least wash their hands and face, if not shower. If showers are not available on site, it is recommended that workers shower and wash their hair immediately upon returning home. Workers' families are at exceptional risk for exposure to lead dust carried home on the worker's clothing or body (McDiarmid & Weaver, 1993); therefore, work clothes should be left or disposed of at the worksite.

Third, abatement proceedings should be carried out with careful attention to containment of the lead dust and fragments that result from the work. Lead-contaminated dust must be painstakingly excluded from nonwork areas (Lange, 1991). This can be done by constructing barriers of 6-mil polyethylene sheeting to isolate living areas and heating/ventilation systems from contaminated areas. In addition, all movable furniture should be removed from the work area, and non-movable furniture should be covered with polyethylene sheeting secured in place with tape. In order to prevent lead-containing dust from settling into cracks in the floor, floor sheeting should be constructed with 6-mil polyethylene sheeting and should extend to the top of the baseboard.

Fourth, after properly trained workers have been enlisted and steps have been taken to protect the workers and contain the work area, actual abatement measures can begin. As discussed above, this may involve replacement of certain building components (e.g., doors, window sills, baseboards), encapsulation, or paint removal. Although the specific procedures and materials that are considered acceptable for encapsulating lead-bearing surfaces vary from region to region, the CDC recommends that the materials be sturdy and prefers that they be attached with both fasteners and adhesives. Frequently used materials include gypsum board, fiberglass mats, vinyl wall coverings, formica, tile, paneling, vinyl or aluminum siding, and newly designed materials specifically for lead containment. Encapsulation of floor surfaces is frequently performed with tile, vinyl flooring, wood, or stone. Standard paint is *not* an acceptable capsulant, nor is any material that will eventually chip, peel, or flake with aging. The removal of intact lead-based paint from a surface and the removal of chalking, peeling, flaking, or otherwise damaged paint is most safely and effectively done by properly trained, protected workers, with one of the following methods: 1) wet hand scraping, with or without use of a heat gun; 2) dry hand scraping of interior surfaces, with or without use of a heat gun; or 3) use of nonflammable chemical strippers that do not contain methylene chloride. As noted above, the following are unsafe means of removing lead-based paint: use of open-flame torches to burn off paint; sanding or grinding paint without the use of an industrial HEPA vacuum; and uncontained waterblasting, sandblasting, or dry-scraping without concomitant misting.

Fifth, following abatement procedures, the abatement area must be cleaned thoroughly. Lead-based paint removal always generates a large amount of lead-containing dust, and paint removal from most surfaces leaves a residue that may not be visible but nevertheless contains toxic levels of lead. Consequently, before abated surfaces can be repainted, they should be vacuumed with an industrial HEPA vacuum filtration device (HEPA filtration is capable of filtering 0.3-μm particles with 99.97% efficiency). After HEPA-vacuuming, surfaces should be scrubbed with a high-phosphate detergent such as trisodium phosphate. To ensure that airborne lead has had time to settle, a second cleanup should be conducted no sooner than 1 hour after the initial cleanup has been completed and should again consist of HEPA-vacuuming followed by wet-cleaning with a high-phosphate detergent. Abated surfaces can then be repainted or, in the case of floors, recoated. Following repainting or recoating, surfaces should again be HEPA-vacuumed, wet-washed, and HEPA-vacuumed for a final time. At this point, a surface wipe test should be conducted to verify that abatement has reduced lead to acceptable levels. Although there are presently no federal dust lead standards for determining when an abated dwelling can be reoccupied, HUD has cited standards used by the states of Maryland and Massachusetts and recommended them as tentative clearance criteria until new guidelines are issued. These standards are as follows: 200 μg/ft^2 for floors, 500 μg/ft^2 for window sills, and 800 μg/ft^2 for window wells (Davis et al., 1993; Keck, 1990; U.S. Department of Housing and Urban Development, 1990b). It should be pointed out that these HUD guidelines were determined primarily on the basis of practicality rather than on any assessment of health impact and that they are currently undergoing revision.

Sixth, lead-based paint abatement often generates a large amount of waste that must be disposed of properly. Determination must be made on a case-by-case basis as to whether the concentration of lead in the waste is high enough to result in classification of the waste as hazardous material. In instances where the waste does not meet the definition of hazardous material, it should be wrapped or bagged, sealed in plastic, and then disposed of in a landfill. Because incineration of lead waste results in the dispersal of lead into the air, this is an unacceptable means of disposal. When classified as hazardous, lead waste must be handled by a licensed transporter. Once abatement has been completed and the waste material disposed of properly, a final reinspection should be carried out to verify the effectiveness of the abatement process.

There seems to be little doubt that lead-based paint abatement, when properly conducted, should result in significant reduction of blood lead concentrations in children with lead poisoning who live in the abated dwellings. In fact, evidence suggests that even comparatively nonaggressive lead-based paint hazard remediation can have a positive impact (Staes, Matte, Copley, Flanders, & Binder, 1994). Nevertheless, abatement of lead-based paint as described above is an extremely costly enterprise and one for which public funds have not been forthcoming on as large a basis as necessary. In fact, a number of proposals for making deleading more economically feasible have been suggested. Perhaps one of the more creative proposals was the suggestion by Needleman (1989) to train unemployed individuals to delead and rehabilitate houses under safe conditions and to allow such labor to be used to purchase equity in the housing.

Another approach, proposed in New York City, is intended to allow multitiered, economical lead hazard reduction, which would result in "the greatest benefit to the largest number of children in the shortest period of time" (Goodman et al., 1993, p. 242). Although recognized as a temporary strategy in some cases, the plan involves an initial risk assessment based primarily on lead dust measurements. A risk level is then assigned to one of three possible categories, based on the HUD dust clearance criteria discussed above. A Level 1 hazard would be a dwelling with dust lead samples less than the HUD clearance values; the Level 1 response would entail wet-scraping of defective painting, followed by wet-cleaning and HEPA-vacuuming and repainting of the affected area. A Level 2 hazard involves a lead dust sample up to five times greater than the HUD clearance levels; a Level 2 response comprises the steps taken for a Level 1 response plus removal of lead paint from friction surfaces as well as encapsulation of interior sills and other chewable surfaces. A Level 3 hazard is defined as a dwelling in which any dust sample exceeds five times the HUD clearance values *or* a dwelling that houses a child with a blood lead concentration of ≥ 20 μg/dL. The Level 3 response involves the steps taken for a Level 2 response plus replacement of windows and all deteriorated substrates, sealing of floors, and encapsulation or replacement of all surfaces that cannot be made intact. Although this approach does not result in complete or permanent lead hazard reduction in many instances and would require ongoing monitoring, Goodman et al. (1993) suggest that it is an effective means of directing scarce resources to the dwellings with the greatest hazards.

Dust

Dust control can contribute significantly to a reduction in childhood lead exposure. For example, wet-mopping and frequent hand washing have been shown to reduce blood lead concentrations in children with elevated blood lead levels (Charney, Kessler, Farfel, & Jackson, 1983), although these cannot be viewed as a long-term solution in the absence of abatement of the source of the lead in the dust. Nevertheless, a 1994 study suggests that sustained reductions of dust lead hazards *can* be achieved in comprehensively abated dwellings (Farfel, Chisolm, & Rohde, 1994). Details of lead-contaminated dust abatement procedures are included in the section above on lead-based paint abatement and the section below on lead-contaminated soil abatement.

Soil

The lead content in soil comes primarily from three sources: lead-based paint that has chalked or peeled from a nearby building, leaded gasoline, and industrial sources. Although lead emissions from gasoline have been largely eliminated, it is estimated that 4–5 million metric tons of lead from gasoline remains in dust and soil (Agency for Toxic Substances and Disease Registry, 1988). Furthermore, although industrial sources contribute to soil lead in only certain locations (Galvin, Stephenson, Wlodarczyk, Loughran, & Waller, 1993), it is common for soil adjacent to houses painted with lead-based paint on the exterior to be contaminated with lead (Mielke et al., 1983). In addition, because lead is not biodegradable, the lead present in soil does not decay and therefore remains a threat indefinitely.

When to Abate   The quantity of lead present in soil is variable from region to region and even within a region. According to the EPA, soil within 25 m of roadways often has lead levels as much as 2,000 ppm greater than intrinsic levels, with some soils having concentrations as much as 10,000 ppm. Soil adjacent to houses that are painted on the exterior with lead-based paint may also have lead levels >10,000 ppm (U.S. EPA, 1986). Not surprisingly, several studies have demonstrated a relationship between concentration of lead in soil and children's blood lead concentrations (Charney, Sayre, & Coulter, 1980; Mielke et al., 1983; Stark, Quah, Meigs, & Delousie, 1982). Although many health departments use the EPA Office guidelines discussed above with regard to soil lead levels (≥400 ppm as a trigger concentration effecting cleanup efforts in areas frequented by children), no commonly accepted standard or enforceable level currently exists. In 1989, the New Jersey Department of Health adopted the following recommendations based on the known dose–response relationships of lead in soil and blood lead in children:

1. A maximum permissible level of 250 ppm of lead in soil in areas without grass cover and repeatedly used by children below age 5 years
2. A maximum permissible level of 600 ppm of lead in soil in areas repeatedly used by children below 12 years of age (This level would contribute no more than 5 µg/dL to the blood lead level in children.)
3. A maximum permissible level of 1,000 ppm of lead in soil in areas such as industrial parks or along streets and in other areas not frequented by children (Madhavan, Rosenman, & Shehata, 1989)

Because these recommendations were instituted prior to the most recent CDC guidelines, it seems likely that the levels may eventually require downward adjustment because even a contribution of 5 µg/dL to the blood lead concentration may represent a significant risk to a child with other possible lead exposures.

Abatement Procedures A number of approaches have been used to reduce exposure to lead-contaminated soil:

1. In instances where soil lead concentrations are not extremely elevated (some agencies use 10,000 ppm as a cutoff), hazard reduction may include complete covering of the soil with concrete, asphalt, gravel (to a minimum depth of 4 inches), mulch (to a minimum depth of 6 inches), sod, new grass, or other impassable greenery.
2. Diluting wet or damp soil (to avoid dust formation) by roto-tilling with lead-free soil and/or mulch to reduce the concentration of lead in the soil to an acceptable level (frequently <400 ppm), followed by covering the soil with lead-free soil to a depth of at least 3 inches
3. Complete excavation, removal, and replacement of lead-contaminated soil with uncontaminated soil

To date, there are few data demonstrating the effectiveness of any of these techniques for soil abatement in reducing blood lead concentrations in children. A study in Boston examined the effectiveness of reducing the lead content of soil in urban neighborhoods with a high incidence of childhood lead poisoning and high soil lead levels by removing a 15-cm layer of topsoil and replacing it with 20 cm of uncontaminated soil (Weitzman et al., 1993). Although this intervention did result in a modest decline in blood lead levels (mean decline = 2.44 µg/dL), the investigators concluded that the magnitude of the reduction was not sufficient to justify this method of abatement for the majority of urban children with low-level lead exposure in the United States. Techniques for reducing the bioavailability of lead in soil are currently under study (Rabinowitz, 1993), although the clinical applicability remains to be determined.

Water

Data regarding the contribution that lead-contaminated water makes to the overall incidence of lead poisoning are conflicting. For example, a study in London, Ontario, Canada, found no evidence that children living in an area serviced by lead pipes had a higher blood lead level than children living in other areas not serviced by lead pipes, even when adjusted for such factors as gender, year of lead test, and census tract (Alder, Dillon, Loomer, Poon, & Robertson, 1993). Yet, according to estimates by the EPA, approximately 2% of children in the United States who do not live in housing with deteriorating lead-based paint and who are not exposed to high levels of lead in the soil nevertheless have blood lead levels above 10 µg/dL (U.S. EPA, 1990). It is further estimated that if all lead in drinking water were eliminated, this percentage would be reduced to 1.4%.

When to Abate   Although the EPA has declared 15 µg/L as the maximum contaminant action level, municipalities vary regarding the required action to be taken for concentrations in excess of that level. In Rhode Island, for example, when flushed samples have lead concentrations of 5–14 µg/L, the Environmental Lead Management Plan includes requirements for both flushing and for reducing water intake to 0.5 L per person per day. However, when the lead concentration in a flushed sample is 15–100 µg/L, the plan requires prohibition of intake. Only when the lead concentration exceeds 100 µg/L is active lead hazard reduction required.

Abatement Procedures   Reduction of lead in drinking water requires a sequential approach in many cases. When elevated levels have been detected, the concentration of lead in the public water supply servicing the dwelling (if the dwelling is so supplied) should be determined. Alternatively, if the dwelling is serviced by a well, the lead content of water within the well should be measured. In instances when municipal water supplies contain elevated levels of lead, public water suppliers may take steps to reduce the corrosivity of the water and thus the amount of lead that leaches into the drinking water.

On an individual household basis, there are several practical measures that can help reduce the amount of lead in drinking water: using only water from the cold water tap for drinking and cooking (because hot water dissolves lead more easily from pipes and plumbing fixtures), using fully flushed water for drinking and cooking, and maintaining plumbing in good working order. Active removal of lead from drinking water can be performed with reverse osmosis or distillation units; carbon and cartridge water filters do not remove lead from water. In its simplest form, a reverse osmosis system consists of a pump, a membrane, and a flow regulator on the wastewater. There may also be a sediment prefilter to reduce fouling of the reverse osmosis membrane. Distillation devices remove lead by boiling the water and condensing the steam. Many impurities are left behind, resulting in nearly contaminant-free water. Although these units frequently produce water with a somewhat bland taste, distillation is capable of removing approximately 99% of the lead from water.

CONCLUSIONS

Our knowledge of the health effects of lead has grown exponentially since the early 1970s. Unfortunately, our understanding of the most appropriate means to deal with the issue of lead in the environment has grown at a much slower pace. There continues to be a need for refinement of current abatement methods and the development of new ones that are not only effective but cost-effective as well. As Davis et al. (1993) pointed out,

> Ultimately, a substantial societal commitment is likely to be essential if the manifold dimensions of the lead problem are to be successfully addressed. Much has been accomplished thus far, but much remains to be done before we can claim to have eliminated lead as an environmental health issue. (p. 24)

REFERENCES

Agency for Toxic Substances and Disease Registry. (1988). *The nature and extent of lead poisoning in children in the United States: A report to Congress*. Atlanta: U.S. Department of Health and Human Services, Public Health Service.

Alder, R., Dillon, J., Loomer, S., Poon, H., & Robertson, J. (1993). An analysis of blood lead data in clinical records by external data on lead pipes and age of household. *Journal of Exposure Analysis and Environmental Epidemiology, 3*(3), 299–314.

Amitai, Y., Brown, M.J., Graef, J.W., & Cosgrove, E. (1991). Residential deleading: Effects on the blood lead levels of lead-poisoned children. *Pediatrics, 88*(5), 893–897.

Annest, J. (1983). Trends in the blood lead levels of the U.S. population. In M. Rutter & R. Jones (Eds.), *Lead versus health* (pp. 33–58). New York: John Wiley & Sons.

Centers for Disease Control (CDC). (1985). *Preventing lead poisoning in young children: A statement by the Centers for Disease Control*. Atlanta: U.S. Department of Health and Human Services, Public Health Service.

Centers for Disease Control (CDC). (1991). *Preventing lead poisoning in young children: A statement by the Centers for Disease Control*. Atlanta: U.S. Department of Health and Human Services, Public Health Service.

Charney, E., Kessler, B., Farfel, M., & Jackson, D. (1983). Childhood lead poisoning: A controlled trial of the effect of dust control measures on blood lead levels. *New England Journal of Medicine, 309*, 1089–1093.

Charney, E., Sayre, J., & Coulter, M. (1980). Increased lead absorption in inner city children: Where does the lead come from? *Pediatrics, 65*, 226–231.

Chisolm, J.J. (1986). Removal of lead paint from old housing: The need for a new approach. *American Journal of Public Health, 76*, 236–237.

Chisolm, J.J., Mellits, E., & Quaskey, S. (1985). The relationship between the level of lead absorption in children and the age, type, and condition of housing. *Environmental Research, 38*, 31–45.

Davis, J., Elias, R., & Grant, L. (1993). Current issues in human lead exposure and regulation of lead. *Neurotoxicology, 14*, 15–27.

Farfel, M.R., Chisolm, J.J., Jr., & Rohde, C.A. (1994). The longer-term effectiveness of residential lead paint abatement. *Environmental Research, 66*(2), 217–221.

Farfel, M., Lees, P., Rohde, C., Lim, B., Bannon, D., & Chisolm, J. (1994). Comparison of a wipe and a vacuum collection method for the determination of lead in residential dusts. *Environmental Research, 65*, 291–301.

Galvin, J., Stephenson, J., Wlodarczyk, J., Loughran, R., & Waller, G. (1993). Living near a lead smelter: An environmental health risk assessment in Boolaroo and Argenton, New South Wales. *Australian Journal of Public Health, 17*(4), 373–378.

Goodman, A., Shultz, H., Klitzman, S., Kimmelblatt, M., & Spadaro, W. (1993). Preventing lead poisoning in New York City: Priorities for lead abatement in housing. *Bulletin of the New York Academy of Medicine, 70*(3), 236–250.

Grondona, C. (1993). Lead revisited: A case study on lead exposed painters. *AAOHN Journal, 41*(1), 33–38.

Housing and Community Development Act of 1992, PL 102-550. (October 28, 1992). Title 42, U.S.C. §§ 1437 et seq.: *U.S. Statutes at Large, 106*, 3672–4097.

Keck, J. (1990). Abatement of lead-based paint. In *A new look at lead toxicity: Conference on Childhood Lead Toxicity* (pp. 20–24). Fort Washington, PA: McNeil Consumer Products Co.

Lange, J. (1991). A suggested air standard for lead to protect the public during lead abatement activities. *Medical Hypotheses, 36*, 211–212.

Madhavan, S., Rosenman, K., & Shehata, T. (1989). Lead in soil: Recommended maximum permissible levels. *Environmental Research, 49*, 136–142.

McDiarmid, M., & Weaver, V. (1993). Fouling one's own nest revisited. *American Journal of Industrial Medicine, 24*, 1–9.

Mielke, H., Anderson, J., Berry, K., Mielke, P., Chaney, R., & Leech, M. (1983). Lead concentrations in inner-city soils as a factor in the child lead problem. *American Journal of Public Health, 73*, 1366–1369.

Needleman, H. (1989). The persistent threat of lead: A singular opportunity. *American Journal of Public Health, 79*(5), 643–645.

Que Hee, S., Peace, B., Clark, C., Boyle, J., Bornschein, R., & Hammond, P. (1985). Evolution of efficient methods to sample lead sources, such as house dust and hand dust, in the homes of children. *Environmental Research, 38*(1), 77–95.

Rabinowitz, M. (1993). Modifying soil lead bioavailability by phosphate addition. *Bulletin of Environmental Contamination and Toxicology, 51,* 438–444.

Rabinowitz, M., Leviton, A., Needleman, H., Bellinger, D., & Waternaux, C. (1985). Environmental correlates of infant blood lead levels in Boston. *Environmental Research, 38*(1), 96–107.

Safe Drinking Water Act Amendments, PL 99-339. (June 19, 1986). Title 42, U.S.C. §§ 300f et seq.: *U.S. Statutes at Large, 100,* 642–667.

Schwartz, J., & Levin, R. (1991). The risk of lead toxicity in homes with lead paint hazard. *Environmental Research, 54,* 1–7.

Staes, C., Matte, T., Copley, C., Flanders, D., & Binder, S. (1994). Retrospective study of the impact of lead-based paint hazard remediation on children's blood lead levels in St. Louis, Missouri. *American Journal of Epidemiology, 139*(10), 1016–1026.

Stark, A., Quah, R., Meigs, J., & Delousie, E. (1982). The relationship of environmental lead to blood lead levels in children. *Environmental Research, 27,* 372–383.

U.S. Department of Housing and Urban Development (HUD). (1990a). *Comprehensive and workable plan for the abatement of lead-based paint in privately owned housing: Report to Congress.* Washington, DC: Author.

U.S. Department of Housing and Urban Development (HUD). (1990b, September). *Lead-based paint: Interim guidelines for hazard identification and abatement in public and Indian housing, Official revised edition.* Washington, DC: Office of Public and Indian Housing.

U.S. Environmental Protection Agency (EPA). (1975). National interim primary drinking water regulations. *Federal Register, 40,* 59,566.

U.S. Environmental Protection Agency (EPA). (1986). *Air quality criteria for lead.* No. EPA-600/8-83-028aF-dF. Washington, DC: Office of Health and Environmental Assessment, Environmental Criteria and Assessment Office.

U.S. Environmental Protection Agency (EPA). (1989/1990). *Interim guidance and supplement to interim guidance on establishing soil lead cleanup levels at Superfund sites.* Washington, DC: Office of Solid Waste and Emergency Response, Directives 9355.4-02 and 9355.4-02A.

U.S. Environmental Protection Agency (EPA). (1990). *Strategy for reducing lead exposures.* Washington, DC: Author.

U.S. Environmental Protection Agency (EPA). (1991). Maximum contaminant level goals and national primary drinking water regulations for lead and copper. *Federal Register, 56,* 26,460–26,564.

Weitzman, M., Aschengrau, A., Bellinger, D., Jones, R., Hamlin, J., & Beiser, A. (1993). Lead-contaminated soil abatement and urban children's blood lead levels. *Journal of the American Medical Association, 269*(13), 1647–1654.

Zedd, H., Walker, Y., Hernandez, J., & Thomas, R. (1993). Lead exposures during shipboard chipping and grinding paint-removal operations. *American Industrial Hygiene Association Journal, 54*(7), 392–396.

10

LEAD-BASED
PAINT LEGISLATION

Stephanie Pollack
Jeanne M. Solé

A s the adverse effects of lead poisoning, even at low blood lead concentrations, are becoming better understood and accepted, federal and state regulation of lead poisoning prevention, detection, and treatment is increasing. The most comprehensive and important piece of federal legislation is the Residential Lead-Based Paint Hazard Reduction Act of 1992 (PL 102-550), popularly known as Title X. As described later in this chapter, Title X provides for federal regulation of the private industry that will evaluate and control lead-based paint hazards in housing, imposes control requirements in federally assisted housing, and authorizes grants to cities and states to help fund primary prevention. In addition, several federal agencies have published standards and guidelines with respect to blood lead screening and lead-based paint hazard identification and control, but, except in the case of programs funded in whole or in part by the federal government, legal requirements in these areas are established by the individual states. In general, then, states (or sometimes counties or cities) remain primarily responsible for regulating critical aspects of primary and secondary prevention ranging from screening and case management of poisoned children to requirements for controlling lead-based paint hazards in housing.

Although Title X does not directly govern many aspects of state-level regulation of lead, it sets an important overall direction by focusing environmental remediation efforts on lead-based paint, which was applied to homes extensively prior to 1950 and more sporadically until 1978. Hazards arising from lead-based paint include dust and bare residential soil contaminated by paint, deteriorated paint, and some types of intact paint that present exposure concerns. Recent federal and state enactments recognize that, because lead additives have been eliminated from gasoline, lead-based paint hazards in residential properties are the most significant source of childhood lead poisoning.

Lead laws are increasingly addressing a range of topics, including the following:

- Screening of children
- Acceptable methods to conduct lead-based paint hazard identification and control
- Requirements for building owners to control lead-based paint hazards prior to poisoning, commonly referred to as primary prevention
- Environmental intervention when children with elevated blood lead levels are identified
- Training requirements for workers engaged in lead-based paint hazard identification and control
- Disclosure requirements during the sale or lease of residential properties

Certain other topics are also regulated at both the federal and state levels but are not discussed in this chapter:

- Particular uses of lead (e.g., prohibitions on the use of lead in gasoline and paint intended for use in residences)
- Lead emissions from stationary sources
- Lead in drinking water
- Worker exposure to lead dust

Legislation and regulations vary considerably from state to state. Whereas some states, such as Massachusetts and Maryland, have enacted comprehensive lead poisoning prevention statutes, other states, such as Indiana and South Dakota, have little lead legislation (Farquhar, 1994). However, even in states where there is little or no legislation relating directly to lead, departments of health may have authority to act pursuant to general authority to maintain public health. Moreover, requirements to control lead-based paint hazards may be inferred by courts from statutes and common-law doctrines relating to negligence, landlord–tenant relationships, and even consumer protection.

Federal and state legal requirements relating to lead poisoning prevention have evolved and will continue to evolve rapidly as additional information is developed about appropriate techniques to identify and control lead-based paint hazards. This chapter thus identifies relevant issues and provides a snapshot of current legal requirements.

SCREENING

Because in most cases lead poisoning involves no immediate discernible symptoms, regular screening of children is a critical component of any comprehensive program to eliminate childhood lead poisoning. The Centers for Disease Control and Prevention (CDC) has recommended universal screening, regular screening must be provided in state "well child" programs funded by Medicaid, and more than half of all states have enacted some form of screening legislation (Farquhar, 1994).

CDC Recommendations

In October 1991, the CDC issued the fourth and most recent revision of "Preventing Lead Poisoning in Young Children" (CDC, 1991), a document setting forth the CDC's recommendations for the prevention of childhood lead poisoning. Although the statements therein are recommendations rather than requirements, they carry behind them the prestige of the CDC, and several states use them as the basis for state-mandated screening requirements.

"Preventing Lead Poisoning in Young Children" recommends the following:

1. That "all children should be screened, unless it can be shown that the community in which these children live does not have a childhood lead poisoning problem" (p. 39). The document points out that, in order to reliably identify the communities that do not have enough of a problem to warrant continued universal screening, a large number or percentage of children must be tested (p. 39).
2. That physicians assess a child's risk for lead exposure during regular office visits starting at 6 months of age. Children at low risk for lead exposure should receive a blood lead test "at 12 months and again, if possible, at 24 months." Children potentially at high risk for lead exposure should be tested when the high risk determination is made (pp. 42–45).
3. That, because erythrocyte protoporphyrin (EP) is not sensitive enough to identify more than a small percentage of children with blood levels between 10 and 25 µg/dL and misses many children with blood lead levels ≥25 µg/dL, measurement of blood lead

levels should replace the EP test as the primary screening method (p. 41).

4. That, although capillary blood samples can be used as an initial screening mechanism, venous blood samples should be required to confirm elevated blood levels (p. 41).

Medicaid Requirements

Pursuant to the Early and Periodic Screening, Diagnosis, and Treatment Program, Medicaid requires states to provide a preventive health program for children (Guthrie & McNulty, 1993). The program must include "[s]creening services which are provided at intervals which meet reasonable standards of medical and dental practice" (Omnibus Budget Reconciliation Act of 1989, 42 U.S.C. § 1396d(r)(1)(A)). Medicaid specifically requires screening services to include "lead blood level assessment appropriate for age and risk factors" (Omnibus Budget Reconciliation Act of 1989, 42 U.S.C. § 1396d(r)(1)(B)(iv)).

Medicaid requirements for blood lead screening are detailed in the *State Medicaid Manual* of the Health Care Financing Administration, the agency responsible for the Medicaid program (Guthrie & McNulty, 1993). The manual states that "all children from 6 months to 72 months are considered at risk and must be screened for lead poisoning" (U.S. Department of Health and Human Services [DHHS], 1993, §5123.2.D.1). It requires that "[b]eginning at six months of age and at each visit thereafter, the provider must...assess the child's risk for exposure" (DHHS, 1993, §5123.2.D.1.a). Low-risk children must receive a blood lead test at 12 and at 24 months of age (DHHS, 1993, §5123.2.D.1.b). High-risk children must receive a blood lead test "when a child is identified as being high risk" (DHHS, 1993, §5123.2.D.1.b).

State Screening Legislation

In response to escalating concern about the prevalence and effects of elevated blood lead levels, states are increasingly enacting screening legislation. Existing state screening legislation includes some or all of the following requirements:

- Mandates for health care providers to screen and/or provide information about screening
- Establishment of the type of test that must be used
- Establishment of the laboratory that must be used
- Mandates for physicians and/or laboratories to report screening results to state departments of health
- Mandates that screening be covered by general health insurance policies

A number of states require health care providers to screen and/or provide information about screening. Three examples are given to illustrate this type of regulation: Rhode Island, Maine, and Vermont. Rhode Island, along with a handful of other states, has enacted mandatory universal screening. Rhode Island law requires physicians to screen children "at the intervals and using the methods" specified by regulation (Lead Poisoning Prevention Act, R.I. Gen. Laws § 23-24.6-7(2) (1991)). To facilitate enforcement of the screening requirement, Rhode Island law requires that upon enrollment child care programs, nursery schools, and kindergartens obtain from a parent or guardian proof that children have been screened (Lead Poisoning Prevention Act, 1993, R.I.).

In contrast, Maine law requires universal access to and information about screening. Maine physicians are required to "advise parents of the availability and advisability of screening their children for lead poisoning" (Lead Poisoning Prevention Act, 1992, Me. Rev. Stat. Ann. tit. 22, § 1317-C.1). However, Maine law does not require physicians to screen all children. Vermont law on screening (An Act Relating to Childhood Lead Poisoning Screening and Lead Hazard Abatement, Vt. Stat. Ann. tit. 18, § 1755(c) (1993)) is something of a hybrid between the Rhode Island and Maine approaches. It requires the department of health to establish guidelines for screening of children and, like the Maine law, requires that

> all health care providers who provide primary medical care shall ensure that parents and guardians of children below the age of six are advised of the availability and advisability of screening and testing their children for lead poisoning. (Vt. Stat. Ann. tit. 18, § 1755(c))

However, mandatory screening similar to that required in Rhode Island is imposed if, after 2 years, the required provision of information to parents does not result in screening of at least 75% of children under the age of 6 years.

A number of states that require screening or the provision of information about screening require their departments of health to issue regulations about acceptable screening methods. Acceptable screening methods are generally, but not always, established by regulation rather than by statute to allow greater flexibility to update legal requirements as more accurate and cost-effective methods of screening are developed.

Increasingly, both the federal government and states have begun regulating laboratories that analyze human fluids or tissues for lead content. Several states require that only state laboratories be used. For example, Rhode Island law requires that all blood samples taken by physicians or other health care providers licensed in Rhode Island, or by licensed, registered, or approved health care facilities in Rhode Island from children under the age of six (6) years for the purpose of screening for blood lead level shall be sent to the state laboratory in the Department of Health for laboratory analysis. (Lead Poisoning Prevention Act, R.I. Gen Laws §§ 23-24.6-7(5))

Other states require only certification of laboratories that conduct analysis of human samples. For example, New Hampshire requires certification of laboratories "performing tests to detect or measure lead in human body fluids or tissues" (Lead Poisoning Prevention and Control Act, N.H. Rev. Stat. Ann. § 130-4:9 (1993)). On the federal level, the CDC operates a voluntary quality control program for laboratories that analyze blood samples, called the Blood Lead Proficiency Testing Program (Guthrie & McNulty, 1993).

A large number of states mandate physicians or laboratories or both to report at least some screening results to state departments of health. According to the National Conference of State Legislatures, 37 states have some form of reporting or state registry (Farquhar, 1994). Some states require reporting of only cases in which lead poisoning is diagnosed or suspected. For example, physicians in Maine must report both known and suspected incidents of poisoning (Lead Poisoning Control Act, 1993, Me.). Others permit departments of health to request more general screening information from health care providers or laboratories. For example, Vermont gives the department of health broad authority to request information from laboratories (An Act Relating to Childhood Lead Poisoning Screening and Lead Hazard Abatement, 1993, Vt.). Finally, a number of states require that lead screening for children be covered by general health insurance policies.

PRIMARY PREVENTION: IDENTIFICATION AND CONTROL OF LEAD-BASED PAINT HAZARDS AND WORKER TRAINING

There is substantial agreement both at the federal and state government levels that improper identification and control of lead-based paint hazards can result in the creation of additional hazards rather than their elimination. Some of the most significant provisions in the Residential Lead-Based Paint Hazard Reduction Act of 1992 (PL 102-550) (Title X) relate to 1) training workers engaged in the identification and control of lead-based paint hazards in residential housing, 2) developing standard definitions of such hazards, and 3) developing guidelines to address them.

The training provisions of Title X apply to lead-based paint hazard activities in most pre-1978 residential housing, both public and private (Residential Lead-Based Paint Hazard Reduction Act of 1992, PL 102-550). (The federal government banned the use of lead-based paint in housing in 1978.) States can adopt stricter standards, so the particular laws and regulations of each individual state should always be consulted before lead-based paint hazard identification or control activities are commenced.

In contrast, federal definitions of lead-based paint hazards are applicable only to states for purposes of Title X, and hazard control guidelines are applicable only to work performed in housing that is either federally owned or receives significant federal assistance. Nonetheless, even where they are not strictly applicable, the concepts, standards, and guidelines that stem from Title X have already significantly affected approaches to lead-based paint hazard control in state legislative and regulatory proceedings and are likely to continue to do so.

Title X is premised on the concept of creating "lead-safe" rather than "lead-free" premises. Thus, Title X focuses on controlling lead-based paint hazards to make pre-1978 homes safe for children rather than providing for the complete removal of lead-based paint in all residential premises. This is because, on the one hand, the complete removal of lead-based paint is viewed as unnecessary to eliminate childhood lead poisoning and, on the other, the cost of complete removal would likely be prohibitive.

Title X sets forth the following broad categories of lead-based paint hazards in homes: deteriorated paint; intact paint on accessible, friction, and impact surfaces; contaminated household dust; and contaminated bare residential soil. The act charges the U.S. Environmental Protection Agency (EPA) to further define the particular levels that constitute a hazard in each broad category. The EPA has issued guidelines further defining hazards and expects to issue final regulations in the fall of 1997.

Because legislatures are moving away from requiring complete removal of lead-based paint, the longevity of hazard control activities becomes important. For example, using thorough and specialized cleanup activities, most lead-contaminated dust can be removed from a dwelling. If no other lead-based paint hazards were present, a home might then be safe for a child to inhabit; however, if the paint that is the source of the dust is not addressed, safe dust levels might last only a few weeks or months. Title X thus creates two categories of lead-based paint hazard control: abatement and interim controls. Both can result in a safe environment; however, interim controls create a safe environment temporarily, and abatement is intended to have more permanent effects.

The focus on lead-based paint hazards rather than on the mere existence of lead-based paint also requires a different type of environmental investigation. Rather than just conducting inspections to determine where lead-based paint is located, "risk assessments" must both identify existing lead-based paint hazards and analyze where and how such hazards are created.

In addition to establishing some fundamental concepts and providing for further definition of lead-based paint hazards, Title X requires the U.S. Department of Housing and Urban Development (HUD) to develop guidelines for lead-based paint hazard identification and control in federally owned housing and housing that receives significant federal assistance. HUD must develop guidelines for risk assessments, inspections, interim controls, and abatement. Although these guidelines are not applicable to entirely private residential homes, they will provide significant technical information on which states can rely in developing statutes and regulations. Guidelines were issued in late 1995.

The training requirements in Title X apply directly to "target housing," which includes all residential homes, both private and public, constructed prior to 1978 except certain housing for elderly or persons with disabilities and no-bedroom dwellings (unless children under 6 years of age live in such units, in which case they are included). The training requirements apply to what Title X defines as lead-based paint activities, which in the case of residential housing include risk assessments, inspections, and abatement, but *not* interim controls. Title X orders the EPA to enact regulations that would

Ensure that individuals engaged in such activities are properly trained
Ensure that training programs are accredited
Ensure that contractors engaged in lead-based paint activities are certified

The regulations must

Include "standards for performing lead-based paint activities, taking into account reliability, effectiveness and safety"
Require that risk assessment, inspection, and abatement be performed by certified workers
Set out requirements for accreditation (Residential Lead-Based Paint Hazard Reduction Act of 1992, § 1021, 15 U.S.C. § 2682)

Title X anticipates that states will implement their own worker training and certification programs, which must be "at least as protective of human health and the environment" (15 U.S.C. § 2684(b)(1)) as federal regulations. If, however, states fail to adopt programs within

2 years after the EPA finalizes its regulations (expected in mid-1996), the federal EPA will run training and certification programs. One difficulty raised by the Title X training and certification requirements is separating those activities that constitute regulated abatement from interim controls and renovation or remodeling activities. Abatement is defined as "any set of measures designed to permanently eliminate lead-based paint hazards in accordance with standards established by the Administrator under this subchapter" (§ 1021, 15 U.S.C. § 2681(1)). Thus, arguably, replacement of a window during the course of energy efficiency home improvements might not constitute abatement, whereas replacement of the same window in order to comply with standards established in Title X would.

Title X begins to address this problem by requiring the EPA to promulgate and disseminate guidelines to control the risk of lead exposure in the course of renovations and remodeling. In addition, Title X requires the EPA to study remodeling and renovation and, within 4 years after enactment of Title X, either require certification of contractors conducting remodeling or renovations or explain why such certification is not appropriate. In the meantime, because Title X sets only minimum training and certification standards, states are free to require training and certification for persons undertaking interim controls and renovation and remodeling work.

PRIMARY PREVENTION: REQUIREMENTS FOR PROPERTY OWNERS

Federal law (Elimination of Lead-Based Paint Hazards in HUD-Associated Housing, 1994; Section 8 Housing Assistance Payments Program, 1994) requires property owners to take certain actions to control lead-based paint hazards in all federally owned target housing or target housing that receives significant federal assistance. In several states, state statutes, regulations, or local ordinances require property owners to control lead-based paint hazards in entirely private housing. Even where no statute exists, "common law" made by courts in lawsuits establishes a "standard of care" to which owners must adhere or risk liability. Generally, children who have been lead poisoned as a result of the existence of lead-based paint hazards in their residence can sue the building owner for damages under common-law negligence theories; poisoned children have also sued with varying degrees of success pursuant to tenant and consumer protection statutes and common-law theories, but such suits are beyond the scope of this chapter and will not be addressed.

Federally Owned or Assisted Housing

Since the early 1970s, federal law has required some control of lead-based paint hazards in federally owned and federally assisted housing even before a child is poisoned (Lead-Based Paint Poisoning Prevention Act of 1971, PL 91-695). In 1992, Title X updated these requirements to incorporate new concepts on lead-based paint hazard identification and control.

In most public housing, Title X requires inspection of a random sample of dwellings and common areas in each project and inspection of each dwelling in a project where lead-based paint hazards are identified. Title X requires abatement in those premises where lead-based paint is found.

In housing that receives project-based federal assistance, Title X requires the secretary of HUD to "establish procedures to eliminate as far as practicable the hazards of lead-based paint poisoning" (§ 1012, 42 U.S.C. § 4822(a)). At a minimum, the statute requires periodic risk assessments and interim controls and sets forth a schedule by which particular percentages of housing must be addressed.

Even though Title X requirements were applicable beginning January 1, 1995, federal regulations have not yet been revised to reflect Title X updates. Instead, existing regulations require only 1) inspections to identify defective paint in applicable federally assisted housing, and covering or removal of any such paint found (Elimination of Lead-Based Paint Hazards in HUD-Associated Housing, 1994); and 2) testing of chewable surfaces for lead-based paint in certain federally assisted housing where a child with an elevated blood lead level resides, and covering or removing any lead-based paint found (e.g., Section 8 Housing Assistance Payments Program, 1994).

Although Title X did not set forth requirements for controlling lead-based paint hazards in entirely private housing, it created a task force to analyze lead-based paint hazard control and financing in such housing. The task force issued its final report in July 1995 (Lead-Based Paint Hazard Reduction and Financing Task Force, 1995).

State Legislation

Several states have enacted legislation and regulations requiring building owners to take steps to control lead-based paint hazards before a child becomes poisoned. Some municipalities have also enacted primary prevention ordinances. Generally, these laws address the following critical questions:

- Who?
- Must do what?

- When?
- With what effect?

In addition, such laws often include specific enforcement provisions. Two such statutes, those of Massachusetts and Maryland, are discussed in further detail to serve as examples.

Massachusetts (Lead Poisoning Prevention and Control Act, Mass., 1994)

Who: Owners of residential premises built before 1978.

Must: Make lead-safe all residential premises where children under 6 years of age reside. Owners may institute interim controls for 2 consecutive years, but then they must conduct abatement. Interim controls and abatement requirements are defined in detail and include requirements for postcontrol cleaning and passing a clearance test for acceptable levels of lead in dust.

When: Owners have the obligation to make residential premises lead-safe whenever a child age 6 or under resides or will reside in the premises.

Effect: Owners who implement interim controls receive a letter of interim control, valid for a year, and owners who implement abatement receive a letter of full compliance, valid indefinitely. Holders of such letters have a duty to ensure that their premises remain in compliance with the requirements for interim control and abatement, respectively. Owners who do not hold letters of interim control or full compliance are "strictly liable" for harm to resident children arising from the failure to comply with the law. That is, in order to win a suit for harm from lead poisoning, a child does not need to prove that the owner knew or should have known that lead-based paint hazards existed in the premises. (See following discussion of common-law negligence.)

If an owner has obtained a letter of interim control or a letter of full compliance, a tenant can no longer use remedies available under the sanitary code (see below). If, however, a sanitary code inspector finds violations in response to a tenant complaint, the owner must pay the cost of the inspection and must correct the violations within 14 days; otherwise, the sanitary code remedies again become available to the tenant.

General liability insurance policies must cover claims for injury or damage from lead poisoning if the owner has a valid letter of interim control or full compliance, unless such injury or damage is the result of gross or willful negligence.

Enforcement: The state Childhood Lead Poisoning Prevention Program and local boards of health (and, in larger cities that have them, housing inspection agencies) have concurrent enforcement responsibility and authority for most aspects of the lead law. These agencies are authorized to use all of the enforcement tools available under the state sanitary code (including issuing administrative orders, levying fines, and bringing civil or criminal judicial proceedings) even before a child is poisoned. Similarly, tenants can use any remedy available under the sanitary code to enforce the lead law, including rent withholding and "repair-and-deduct" remedies. A judge can order that rent withheld be applied to the costs of abatement if the landlord is found not to be acting in good faith.

Maryland   (University of Maryland Law Clinic, 1994)

Who: Owners of residential buildings constructed before 1950 that contain at least one rental unit; the law excludes property owned or operated by government, which is subject to standards at least as stringent, and property that is certified to be lead-free.

Must: Either undertake cleanup or pass a test for lead-contaminated dust. Two standards of cleanup apply: full risk reduction and modified risk reduction. Both involve primarily interim controls rather than abatement. The requirements for full risk reduction and modified risk reduction are defined in detail; full risk reduction is more thorough. At the conclusion of the activities, an inspector must certify that the requirements of the respective reductions have been met.

When: Owners must either pass a clearance test to demonstrate that the levels of lead contamination in dust are acceptable or conduct full risk reduction at the first change in occupancy subsequent to the passage of the law. If risk reduction is selected, it must occur before the next tenant moves in. After this first change in occupancy, owners must either pass a test for lead-contaminated dust or conduct modified risk reduction at each subsequent change in occupancy before the next tenant moves in. Owners must also either pass a test for lead-contaminated dust or perform modified risk reduction in response to a tenant notification of a defect. The law sets forth a schedule to ensure that all properties covered by the law either pass a lead-contaminated dust test or have at least modified risk reduction performed before the year 2004.

Effect: An owner who complies with the law is not liable for damages arising from lead poisoning in his or her property provided that the owner offers relocation and medically necessary treatment pursuant to the law's "qualified offer" provisions. These provisions require a landlord to offer to pay to a poisoned tenant reasonable costs and expenses up to a maximum cap of $9,500 for relocation and $7,500 for medical expenses. Tenants who receive a qualified offer may accept or reject it, but, even if it is rejected, the tenant cannot subsequently sue the owner for the harm occasioned by the lead poisoning.

Insurers must provide coverage for lead hazards to the extent of the qualified offer to owners who comply with the law.

Enforcement: The enforcement provisions of the Maryland Code can be used to enforce the law, but penalties cannot exceed $250 per day.

Common-Law Negligence

Even in states that do not have explicit primary prevention legislation, building owners may have obligations to make rental housing lead-safe pursuant to common-law negligence doctrines or tenant protection statutes. Although the existence of such common-law duties may help to induce rental property owners to control hazards before a child is poisoned, there is usually no mechanism to enforce the obligation until after a poisoning occurs. Then persons injured by an owner's failure to meet his or her obligation can sue to recover damages that result from the failure.

Common-law doctrines on negligence vary from state to state. In general, negligence theories hold that persons have a duty to act reasonably to prevent harm to others. Thus, to win a suit against an owner, a lead-poisoned plaintiff would usually have to show: 1) *duty*—that the owner had a duty to prevent harm; 2) *breach*—that the owner breached his or her duty; 3) *causation*—that, as a result of the breach of duty by the owner, the plaintiff was lead-poisoned; and 4) *harm*—that becoming lead poisoned harmed the plaintiff.

State common law varies with regard to interpretation of what constitutes acting reasonably to prevent harm. One critical issue is whether an owner must actually know that a lead hazard exists before he or she is required to act or whether a plaintiff can demonstrate instead that any prudent owner should have known the danger existed. If it is enough to show that a prudent owner should have known, the next question to be litigated is whether the dangers of lead-based paint are so well understood that a prudent owner of a house built before 1978 should be presumed to know of those dangers. Title X disclosure provisions (see the section on disclosure requirements following) will make it more difficult for owners to argue that they did not know or should not have known about the dangers of lead-based paint; once federal disclosure requirements take effect, purchasers will receive information about lead at the time of purchase and landlords will have to provide renters with such information at the time premises are leased.

Another major issue in lead poisoning litigation involves how far an owner must go to prevent harm in order to fulfill his or her duty to act reasonably. For example, the duty could range from an obligation to completely remove all lead-based paint from the premises to a mere requirement to conduct periodic specialized, thorough cleaning. In the absence of state legislation on this standard-of-care issue, courts may refer to federal standards for interventions in federally owned or assisted properties.

SECONDARY PREVENTION: ENVIRONMENTAL FOLLOW-UP OF LEAD-POISONED CHILDREN

In "Preventing Lead Poisoning in Young Children," the CDC (1991) recommends that in cases where children with blood lead levels of 20 µg/dL and above are identified, environmental investigation and intervention should be initiated within 10 days. Environmental investigation and intervention is also recommended in cases where blood lead levels between 15 and 19 µg/dL persist. As is the case for CDC screening recommendations, the CDC recommendations regarding environmental follow-up do not have the force of law. Instead, direct regulation in this area is relegated to the particular laws of the individual states.

As with most other issues, state requirements for follow-up of poisoning cases vary. Some states mandate very specific responses pursuant to detailed time lines. Other states authorize departments of health to investigate and intervene when a lead-poisoned child is found, but they do not specifically require particular actions in determined time frames. A number of states have requirements for cases involving rental properties more stringent than those applicable to owner-occupied premises. For example, New Hampshire law authorizes but does not order the state's department of health to conduct an environmental investigation in cases where a child with a blood lead level of 20 µg/dL or greater is identified (Lead Poisoning Prevention and Control Act, 1994, N.H.). Once an investigation is initiated, however, the law sets forth detailed requirements for the investigation and, in the case of rental properties, requires the department to order owners to abate any lead-based paint hazards identified.

A significant number of states have not yet enacted legislation that addresses this topic directly. According to the National Conference of State Legislatures, only 13 states have explicit programs for follow-up in the case of a poisoned child (Farquhar, 1994). Even in these states, however, departments of health may have general authority to safeguard the public health, which can be interpreted to allow them to order or conduct some degree of environmental investigation and intervention. However, departments of health tend to be more comfortable ordering significant action when their authority to do so is explicit.

DISCLOSURE REQUIREMENTS

Title X created requirements for disclosure of lead-based paint hazards at the time of sale or rental for all residential properties built before 1978, including wholly private homes (Residential Lead-Based Paint Hazard Reduction Act of 1992, PL 102-550). Title X requires HUD and EPA to develop regulations requiring sellers or lessors to

- Provide potential purchasers or lessees with a lead hazard information pamphlet prepared by EPA
- Disclose the presence of any known lead-based paint, or any known lead-based paint hazards, and provide any available lead inspection reports
- Permit a potential purchaser (but not a prospective renter) 10 days to conduct a risk assessment or inspection

Regulations must also require that any contract for purchase and sale of any interest in target housing include a lead warning statement (as set out in Title X) and a signed statement by the purchaser that he or she

- Has read and understands the warning
- Has received a lead hazard information pamphlet
- Has been given the opportunity to conduct a risk assessment or inspection

Title X provides for the disclosure regulations to take effect October 29, 1995. The final rule has not yet been issued, however. The EPA expects an effective date between spring and winter 1996. A significant number of states have enacted disclosure requirements that apply in advance of the Title X disclosure requirements.

CONCLUSIONS

A patchwork of legislation, regulations, guidelines, and common law governs the detection, treatment, and prevention of lead poisoning as well as compensation of lead poisoning victims. Requirements vary significantly from state to state and are changing rapidly to reflect new information and concerns. Persons acting to prevent lead poisoning should always begin by familiarizing themselves with the most recent federal guidelines and federal and state laws and regulations. Up-to-

date information can be obtained from the EPA Lead Clearinghouse at
1-800-424-LEAD.

REFERENCES

An Act Relating to Childhood Lead Poisoning Screening and Lead Hazard Abatement, Vt. Stat. Ann. tit. 18, § 1755(c) (supp. 1994).

Centers for Disease Control (CDC). (1991). *Preventing lead poisoning in young children* (A statement by the Centers for Disease Control). Atlanta, GA: Author.

Elimination of Lead-Based Paint Hazards in HUD-Associated Housing, 24 C.F.R. § 35.24 (1994).

Farquhar, D. (1994, August). *Lead poisoning prevention: A guide for legislators* (p. xi). Denver, CO: National Conference of State Legislatures.

Guthrie, A.M., & McNulty, M. (1993). *Making the most of Medicaid: State progress in childhood lead poisoning prevention.* Washington, DC: Alliance to End Childhood Lead Poisoning.

Lead-Based Paint Poisoning Prevention Act of 1971, PL 91-695. (January 13, 1971). Title 42, U.S.C. §§ 4801 et seq.: *U.S. Statutes at Large, 84,* 2078–2080.

Lead Poisoning Control Act, Me. Rev. Stat. Ann. tit. 22, § 1317-C.1. (supp. 1994).

Lead Poisoning Prevention and Control Act, Mass. Gen. L. ch. 111, §§ 189A–199B (supp. 1994).

Lead Poisoning Prevention and Control Act, N.H. Rev. Stat. Ann. § 130-A:9 (supp. 1994).

Lead Poisoning Prevention Act, R.I. Gen. Laws § 23–24.6–7 (2) (supp. 1993).

Omnibus Budget Reconciliation Act of 1989, PL 101-239, § 6403(a), Title 42, U.S.C. § 1396d(r)(1)(A) (supp. 1994).

Residential Lead-Based Paint Hazard Reduction Act of 1992, PL 102-550, §§ 1001–61, Title 15, U.S.C. §§ 2681–92; Title 42, U.S.C. §§ 4822–4856 (supp. 1994).

Section 8 Housing Assistance Payments Program—Existing Housing, 24 C.F.R. § 882.109(i)(4) (1994).

University of Maryland Law Clinic. (1994, June 7). *Summary of the Lead Poisoning Prevention Program Act.* Baltimore: Author.

U.S. Department of Health and Human Services (DHHS) Health Care Financing Administration. (1993, October). *State Medicaid Manual* § 5123.2 D.1. (Report No. HCFA-Pub. 45–5). Baltimore: Author.

11

PREVENTION OF
CHILDHOOD LEAD POISONING

Thomas L. Schlenker

Adverse neurologic, behavioral, and growth effects of lead exposure are well documented in infants and young children (Davis
& Svendsgaard, 1987; Dietrich et al., 1987; Faust & Brown, 1987;
McMichael et al., 1988; Needleman & Gastonis, 1990; Shukla, Dietrich, Bornschein, Berger, & Hamilton, 1991). The results of several
studies show that these deficits may persist beyond early childhood
and that long-term consequences are substantial (Baghurst et al.,
1992; Needleman, Schell, Bellinger, Leviton, & Allred, 1990). It has
been estimated that 1.7 million preschool-age children in the United
States have had lead exposures that put them at such risk (Brody et
al., 1994). In addition to individual loss, the societal costs for this
widespread and serious affliction are great. Medical care, remedial
education costs, lifetime lost earnings, and the expense of support-
ing lead poisoning–related social dependency through the social services and prison systems should be factored into total cost. One
authority has speculated that childhood lead poisoning may be
responsible for up to 20% of juvenile delinquency (Needleman,
1990). Prevention of childhood lead poisoning clearly deserves to be
a national priority.

Effective prevention can be thought of as three interrelated activities. *Primary prevention* eliminates lead hazards before exposure can

take place. *Secondary prevention* eliminates or controls lead hazards following detection of exposed children. *Strategic prevention* is the planned long-term effort to eliminate childhood lead poisoning from society and has as its centerpiece nationwide lead-safe housing.

PRIMARY PREVENTION

Primary prevention of childhood lead poisoning is often described with the redundancy "preventing lead poisoning before it occurs." It is thus differentiated from actions that are triggered by blood lead levels that are already elevated. The central aim of primary prevention is to ensure that significant exposure does not occur during the neurologically vulnerable years of early childhood by "preventing entry of the lead source and its removal, reduction or avoidance of contact once present" (Mushak & Crocetti, 1990, p. 125). Fostering lead-safe environments for young children through primary prevention requires the participation of parents, physicians, local public health agencies, the housing industry, governmental rule-making bodies, and many others.

Role of the Federal Government

The extensive use of lead in a multitude of modern products and processes has contaminated much of our environment. The U.S. government has intervened, although at times belatedly, to regulate the use of lead in mining, smelting, manufacturing, construction, and consumer products. From banning lead in shotgun shells to mandating cleanup of Superfund sites, federal law addresses a broad range of potential hazards. Many agencies and branches of government are involved. During the 1980s, the U.S. Food and Drug Administration (FDA) effectively eliminated the use of lead solder in U.S.-made cans containing food or drink (U.S. FDA, 1993). In 1992, the U.S. Environmental Protection Agency (EPA) reduced the allowable concentration of lead in drinking water from 50 µg/dL to 15 µg/dL (Karch and Associates, Inc., 1988; Schlenker, 1989).

The most significant achievement to date is widely considered to be the elimination of lead in gasoline (Annest et al., 1983; Billick, Curran, & Shier, 1980). Introduced in 1923 and not completely banned until 1995, leaded gasoline has added 7 million tons of lead to our surface environment. Over time, the tightening of government regulations and the advent of the catalytic converter have caused the gradual conversion of cars to unleaded gas in the United States. Unleaded fuel technology has greatly improved ambient air quality and is credited with reducing the U.S. population mean blood lead level from 15 µg/dL in 1976 to 6 µg/dL in 1990 (Hayes et al., 1994; Schwartz & Pitcher, 1989).

The use of lead-based paint in the United States has also declined dramatically. Lead was voluntarily removed from most paints in the 1950s. In 1978, approximately 50 years after its ban in Australia and most European countries, lead was officially banned from all residential paint in the United States. Nevertheless, as of this writing and for the foreseeable future, household surfaces painted during the era of leaded paint constitute a major environmental threat to U.S. children. During the period of its use, leaded residential paint introduced 5 million tons of lead into U.S. housing. In 1991, the U.S. Centers for Disease Control and Prevention (CDC) estimated that 14 million homes contained lead hazards and that they were the primary sources of approximately 230,000 annual cases of childhood lead poisoning (CDC, 1988, 1991).

During the 1970s and 1980s, federally funded abatement programs eliminated leaded paint from most public housing in the United States. However, the methods used were so costly that little of the experience is applicable to the private housing market. This is particularly true of low-income rental properties, which house the majority of children who are currently at highest risk for poisoning (U.S. Department of Housing and Urban Development, 1990). In the Residential Lead-Based Paint Hazard Reduction Act of 1992 (PL 102-550), the federal government began the process of implementing market-oriented strategies to eliminate lead hazards from private housing. The act includes provisions to set standards for and determine cost-efficient methods of household lead abatement, to create a new core of trained and licensed abatement workers, to require disclosure of lead hazards on transfer of ownership, and to fund the initial stages of abatement in low-income private housing (Alliance to End Childhood Lead Poisoning, 1993b).

Role of Children's Physicians

Most children in the United States see physicians frequently during the first few years of life. As the U.S. health care system evolves, it is hoped that all children will be guaranteed access to regular medical care. Children's physicians therefore have the best opportunity to intervene during the relatively brief period of early childhood when exposure to lead has its most serious consequences and when effective prevention can take place.

Physicians' knowledge of the phases of early childhood development, linked with awareness of potential sources of lead in and around the home, establishes a rational anticipatory guidance sequence that should be presented to every parent. The danger of exposure to lead hazards advances together with children's ability to explore their environments.

Perinatal Period   Because lead is transferred across the placenta, exposure that would have little or no consequence for the pregnant woman may have devastating effects on the fetus (see also Chapter 7) (Bellinger, Leviton, Waternaux, Needleman, & Rabinowitz, 1987; Dietrich et al., 1987). Inquiry into the potential for maternal exposure to occupational, hobby, home renovation, or other sources of lead during pregnancy should be a universal element of prenatal care. Also, during the newborn period, there are potential dangers in the home that merit discussion with parents at or before birth. Renovations, including getting a home ready for the new baby, may involve hazardous methods or inadequate cleanup that puts newborns at risk (Amitai, Brown, Graef, & Cosgrove, 1991; Marino et al., 1990). The physician should inquire about such activities and, when appropriate, assist the parents in contacting the local public health agency for guidance.

Formula-fed infants can be exposed to significant amounts of lead when the water used to prepare their formula comes through water pipes that are made of lead or joined by lead solder such as those commonly found in older housing (Shannon & Graef, 1992). Explicit bottle-feeding instructions that warn against preparing formula with hot water taken directly from the tap (hot water leaches lead out of the piping) along with instructions to flush and discard first morning tap water (lead accumulates in water that rests in pipes overnight) will avoid this potential exposure.

Early Childhood Development   At about 6–9 months of age, as they learn to crawl, most infants graduate from the crib to the wide open spaces of the living room rug and kitchen floor. Because of their natural propensity to mouth whatever is in their path, crawling infants are doubly exposed to lead-laden dust, paint chips, and other objects that may be found on floors.

When infants learn to stand and walk by holding on to chairs, tables, and window sills, they gain access to chewable surfaces that may be covered with lead paint. The highest concentrations of lead-containing dust and debris are found on window sills and wells, a favorite play site of toddlers. As children gain skill in walking, they are able to visit less traveled areas of the home such as porches, basements, and spare rooms, where even greater lead hazards may exist. Thus, increased vigilance in maintaining a clean and tidy house and common-sense restrictions on where infants and toddlers are allowed to roam should be the order of the day.

When the weather permits, toddlers are often allowed to play out-of-doors. Their play may not be fully supervised and can be perilous for a number of reasons. Outdoor paint and the flakes, chips, and dust that weathering produces often have high concentrations of lead. Such paint debris falls onto the ground adjacent to houses—a preferred site of play for this age group, which typically revels in dirt and has yet to outgrow the mouthing behaviors of infancy. The fact that elevated lead levels are most prevalent among the toddler age group and occur most frequently during late summer has been attributed to outdoor play (Mahaffey, Annest, Roberts, & Murphy, 1982). Parents who anticipate this developmental stage can avoid exposing their children to outdoor lead hazards by using well-placed sod, bushes, and sandboxes filled with clean sand and by appropriately scheduling and implementing repairs of siding, porches, and so forth. Even though older preschool-age children are at decreased risk, studies of urban populations show a fairly high prevalence of lead poisoning through 3 years of age (Brown et al., 1990; Schaffer, Szilagyi, & Weitzman, 1994).

Environmental Risk Assessment Attention to early childhood development must be complemented by knowledge of potential sources of lead in children's environments. Even though physicians generally do not visit patients in their homes, specific information on household lead hazards can be obtained and valuable anticipatory guidance can be delivered as a part of routine in-office well-baby exams.

Physicians should specifically inquire about the age of the family home. Structures built after 1970 are unlikely to contain lead paint, whereas older dwellings, particularly those built before 1950, can be expected to contain substantial amounts of lead. The condition of painted surfaces, inside and out, is key. A brief, structured questionnaire proposed by the CDC and modified by others has been widely used (Binns, LeBailly, Poncher, Kinsella, & Saunders, 1994; Centers for Disease Control, 1988; Nordin, Rolnick, & Griffin, 1994; Tejeda, Wyatt, Rostek, & Solomon, 1994) (Table 1). (See Chapter 4.)

Guidance on the correct preparation of infant formula should be augmented by admonition against allowing food to sit in open metal containers (lead in solder may leach into food when exposed to air)

Table 1. Assessing the risk of high-dose exposure to lead: Sample questionnaire

Does your child

1. Live in or regularly visit a house with peeling or chipping paint built before 1960? This could include a day care center, preschool, or the home of a babysitter or a relative.
2. Live in or regularly visit a house built before 1960 with recent, ongoing, or planned renovation or remodeling?
3. Have a brother or sister, housemate, or playmate being followed or treated for lead poisoning (i.e., blood lead ≥15 µg/dL)?
4. Live with an adult whose job or hobby involves exposure to lead?
5. Live near an active lead smelter, battery recycling plant, or other industry likely to release lead?

and storing liquids in ceramic containers (acidic liquids like fruit juices absorb lead from inadequately fired ceramics) (Mahaffey, 1983; Smith, Beller, & Middaugh, 1992).

It is necessary to identify the occupations of all adults in the household. Mining, smelting, foundry work, welding, radiator repair, battery manufacture and recycling, highway and bridge painting, indoor firearms practice, and housing renovation may expose workers to lead dust that can be brought home on hands, hair, shoes, and clothing. Geographic proximity to a mine or smelter is also of concern (Landrigan & Baker, 1981; Landrigan et al., 1975). Hobbies such as stained glass window making, ceramics, firearms, and the making of lead toys, ammunition, or fishing weights are also potential hazards (Landrigan, 1982; Schlenker, 1992a).

Some children may get exposure from chewing on imported toys colored with lead paint or lead-containing plastics. Lead has also been identified in imported crayons. Some traditional folk medicines and cosmetics of Asia and Latin America to which children can be exposed contain up to 80% lead by weight (Markowitz et al., 1994; Trotter, 1990).

Poor nutrition may stimulate pica. In addition, iron and calcium deficiency states appear to increase absorption across the gut and retention in major organs, especially bone, of the similar cationic lead molecule (Mahaffey, 1981). Counsel on appropriate nutrition for young children, routine screening for iron deficiency anemia, and prescription of iron and calcium supplements as indicated are important elements in the primary prevention of lead poisoning (CDC, 1988) (Table 2).

Role of Local Public Health Agencies

Local public health agencies vary a great deal with respect to the expertise and capacity of their primary prevention programs. At a minimum, health departments should be able to appropriately educate the populations they serve. Exceeding the minimum, many departments have given lead poisoning prevention priority status and have developed an array of primary prevention activities that effectively fill the gap between physician anticipatory guidance and federal government regulation.

Table 2. Major sources of iron and calcium

Iron	Calcium
Liver	Milk
Fortified cereal	Yogurt
Cooked legumes	Cheese
Spinach	Cooked greens

Perhaps the most essential primary prevention activity of public health authorities is to direct attention to children at highest risk for lead poisoning by the ongoing analysis of local population and housing characteristics. Based on such analyses, public health's outreach capacity can be employed to visit high-risk families in their homes in order to educate, inspect, and offer assistance on lead hazard remediation on-site. Public health fieldwork may also reveal non–housing-related lead hazards such as industrial point sources or hazardous cultural practices (e.g., use of lead-containing traditional medicines or cosmetics) that can be addressed proactively.

Relative to housing regulation, health departments customarily have statutory responsibility for enforcing that portion of the housing code that relates to public health and safety. Within the limits allowed by local resources, both the condition of housing and the processes of construction and remodeling can be forced to conform to standards for abatement and maintenance. By providing education and support to homeowners and renovators as well as assessing penalties against those who do not comply with standards, health departments protect the public against the creation of additional lead hazards that can arise from dangerous work practices (Farfel & Chisolm, 1990).

Standards of abatement as well as provisions for their enforcement should be detailed either by city ordinance or by state statute. In many instances, the public health authority will be required to lead the effort to create or substantially revise the laws. Similarly, where qualified abatement contractors are lacking, the public health authority may take the lead in providing for appropriate training, certification, and deployment of workers in this rapidly growing industry. Finally, when needed lead hazard remediation is blocked by lack of funds or adverse housing markets, sources of subsidy may be sought through local philanthropic organizations and individuals, national foundations, or programs of the federal government.

SECONDARY PREVENTION

Secondary prevention of lead poisoning refers to actions that take place after elevated blood lead levels in children have been identified. The goal is to reduce individual lead burden through changes in nutrition, behavior, and environment. Currently, the CDC has set <10 µg/dL as the target level for blood lead in children (CDC, 1988).

Effective secondary prevention depends on mass screening of children for elevated blood lead levels (see Chapter 4). This ex post facto approach has been criticized by some as being a poor substitute for primary prevention and analogous to the tradition of using asphyxiated canaries to warn miners of impending danger. Nevertheless, under the present circumstances in the United States, in which millions of children are exposed to lead, secondary prevention is essential to targeting limited resources to those who are most in need.

It is also important to consider that much is unknown about the toxicology of lead. Although there is no doubt that an increased body burden of lead in infants and young children results in serious and long-term neurologic disabilities, there is an incomplete understanding of the mechanism by which this occurs. The measure used to correlate with neurologic disability by the famous Port Pirie, Australia, studies was average blood lead level calculated from several point-in-time specimens (Baghurst et al., 1992; McMichael et al., 1988). Needleman's groundbreaking study in Somerville, Massachusetts, in the 1970s used lead in teeth as its measure—also a reflection of exposure over time (Needleman et al., 1979, 1990).

Thus, it is conceivable that there may be a threshold of sustained exposure required for adverse outcome. If this is true, then it follows that children with brief low-level elevations of blood lead who are promptly detected and protected from further exposure can escape harm. Secondary prevention, therefore, is much more than an expediency dictated by limited resources. It is first and foremost a practical and necessary strategy to prevent sustained lead hazard exposure in large numbers of children. Although the effectiveness and cost efficiency of most secondary prevention measures are yet to be established, studies on the relative value of interventions from education to complete environmental abatement are beginning to accumulate (Kimbrough, LeVois, & Webb, 1994; Staes, Matte, Copley, Flanders, & Binder, 1994; Weitzman et al., 1993). One hopes that this research will constitute the basis for rational approaches to prevention.

Role of Children's Physicians

For most physicians, secondary prevention begins with office-based screening. In many areas of the United States, blood lead measurements should be obtained on all children 6 months to 6 years of age. In some areas, targeted screening may be the more reasonable approach. Physician responses are dictated by individual blood lead levels and should correspond to the "multitier" schedule of the CDC (Centers for Disease Control, 1991) (Table 3).

Blood lead levels at ≥15 µg/dL alert physicians to children who have experienced some exposure to lead and serve as a guide to individualized childhood behavior/home environment discussions with parents. The discussions should cover the same points addressed in primary prevention, but in greater detail and with a heightened sense of urgency. Child-specific blood lead levels help physicians focus on those children who are most in need while making parents more receptive to the guidance offered.

Table 3. Class of child and recommended action according to blood lead measurement

Class	Blood lead concentration (µg/dL)	Action
I	≤9	Low risk for high-dose exposure: Rescreen as described in text. High risk for high-dose exposure: Rescreen as described in text.
IIA	10–14	Rescreen as described in text. If many children in the community have blood lead levels ≥10, community interventions (primary prevention activities) should be considered by appropriate agencies.
IIB	15–19	Rescreen as described in text. Take a history to assess possible high-dose sources of lead. Educate parents about diet, cleaning, etc. Test for iron deficiency. Consider environmental investigation and lead hazard abatement if levels persist.
III	20–44[a]	Conduct a complete medical evaluation. Identify and eliminate environmental lead sources.
IV	45–69[a]	Begin medical treatment and environmental assessment and remediation within 48 hours
V	≥70[a]	Begin medical treatment and environmental assessment and remediation *immediately.*

Adapted from Centers for Disease Control (1991).
[a]Based on confirmatory blood lead level.

In most communities, physicians provide direct lead poisoning guidance to many more families than health departments are capable of reaching. Thus, physician-guided prevention, even relative to environmental maintenance and repair, has great potential for doing good. Moreover, physician-guided prevention is the only professional intervention that most children with lower-level exposure will receive.

For blood lead levels of ≥20 µg/dL or those that persist ≥15 µg/dL, physicians should involve the local public health agency for inspection, risk assessment, and assistance to families in their homes. Although the public and private health sectors need to work in concert, physicians should maintain continuity of clinical care by regularly monitoring blood lead levels until levels of ≤9 µg/dL are achieved.

Role of Local Public Health Agencies

Screening Effective secondary prevention requires that local public health authorities set the framework for and ensure the implementation of appropriate lead poisoning screening. If universal screening is indicated, then local public health officials must ensure that it is appropriately carried out in the private and public sectors (Schlenker, 1992b; Schlenker, Fritz, Murphy, & Shepeard, 1994). If targeted screening is indicated, then public health authorities must devise approaches that are suitable to local circumstances (Schlenker, Fritz, Mark, et al., 1994).

However, in order to arrive at a suitable approach to screening for any given community, the general prevalence and distribution of lead poisoning must first be estimated. Equations based on housing, socioeconomic, and demographic data extracted from the U.S. Census report and local property tax files can estimate prevalence and map potential risk areas. Over time, actual screening data will supersede the utility of census and tax data, but, until sufficient screenings accumulate, such risk equations can serve as tools for the allocation of resources (Figure 1).

Although the prevalence of lead poisoning among children is best estimated through universal screening, relatively valid prevalence estimates can be made from sufficiently large or randomly selected samples of populations at risk. Aggregate screening data identify the prevalence, distribution, and trends of childhood lead poisoning, which in turn guide programmatic decisions of health departments and strategic decisions of public policy makers. Also, data that are appropriately analyzed, presented, and communicated to physicians reinforce the rationale for screening and help build collaborative public/private relationships.

The CDC currently recommends 20 μg/dL as the blood lead level that should trigger individual case management and environmental intervention. Local public health agencies must necessarily focus such resource-intensive efforts on those children who are most severely affected. Fortunately, the distributions of lead levels within most communities place the majority of children within the safer ranges (Figure 2).

Children with elevated blood lead levels identified through public clinics or reported by the private sector are visited in their homes by health department outreach workers, nurses, and environmental inspectors. They are managed with greater or lesser intensity according to individual blood lead levels and the capacity of the local programs.

Community Outreach Workers Community outreach workers can effectively reach large numbers of children with moderately elevated blood lead levels. Outreach workers should reflect the racial, linguistic, and cultural characteristics of the target population and should be recruited, if possible, from the communities in which they will work. In this way, they are more likely to understand the neighborhoods' operative housing conditions and social dynamics. They are also more likely to gain access to the homes and ultimately the trust of high-risk families. With training and experience, community outreach workers can become expert in the practical aspects of lead poisoning prevention.

Community outreach workers generally meet families in their homes to inform them of their children's blood lead levels, explain

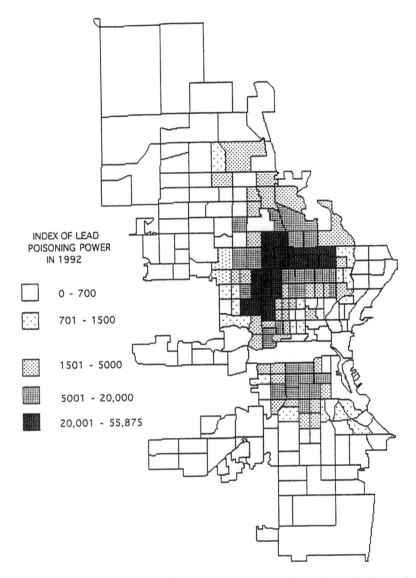

INDEX OF LEAD
POISONING POWER
IN 1992

☐ 0 - 700

▨ 701 - 1500

▨ 1501 - 5000

▨ 5001 - 20,000

■ 20,001 - 55,875

Figure 1. 1992 index of lead poisoning probability, based on 0.91 correlation with number of cases of >25 μg/dL Pb found in 1992, per census tract, City of Milwaukee. Index is based on total number of children under 6 years of age × total female households with children × percentage of housing units built before 1940 × number of housing units that are vacant. (From U.S. Census and Milwaukee Master Property File, Milwaukee Health Dept., P. Werner 8/31/93.)

what the levels mean, and discuss behavioral and environmental issues. An abbreviated walk-through inspection of the home is conducted with the parents. During the walk-through, the outreach worker identifies lead hazards and demonstrates appropriate maintenance or

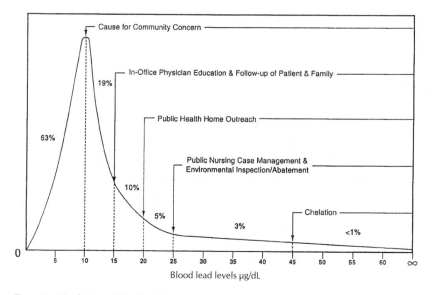

Figure 2.   Distribution of blood lead levels and actions taken for 24,204 screenings, Milwaukee, Wisconsin, 1993. Actions taken are cumulative with ascending levels. (Courtesy of Amy Murphy, MPH, Milwaukee Health Department.)

repair for each hazard. High-energy particulate accumulator vacuum cleaners should be a part of outreach worker equipment, along with mops, buckets, sponges, high-phosphate cleaner, and tape and cardboard for temporary patching. The outreach worker also assists the parent with appropriate referrals and arranges for follow-up blood lead testing and home visits for the child.

Nursing Care Management   For children with confirmed blood lead levels in the higher ranges, typically >20–25µg/dL, individualized nursing care management is recommended. Experienced public health nurses form the core of most health departments and are especially well suited to coordinate the various components of required care. Nurses perform in-home assessments of the physical, nutritional, and developmental condition of children as well as observe family dynamics and environmental surroundings for factors that may influence risk for lead poisoning. Salient findings are professionally addressed on the spot as well as communicated to physicians, who maintain primacy over the clinical care of the children.

Public health nursing case managers complement and extend the work of clinical physicians. Public health nurses can seek out patients who are lost to follow-up, gather information not otherwise available, and coordinate housing, legal, and social services. Moreover, they often serve as advocates for children who endure particularly difficult environmental or social situations.

Environmental Inspection and Risk Assessment Environmental inspection and risk assessment are essential to determining the sources of lead exposure for all children with higher blood lead levels (>20–25µg/dL). The levels that trigger environmental intervention differ by community and are usually determined by the numbers of lead-poisoned children and the available resources.

Health department staff trained in the environmental sciences are deployed to inspect the homes of at-risk children identified through screening. Each home is inspected for lead hazards room-by-room, inside and outside. Lead hazards are defined as lead paint debris, lead-containing dirt and dust, and deteriorated lead-covered surfaces that are accessible to young children. Soil, tap water, and other nonpaint sources may also be tested. The presence of lead is determined by a handheld X-ray fluorescence device or by chemical analysis of samples obtained. Other sites that lead-poisoned children frequent are similarly assessed for risk.

Where health departments have such authority, orders to abate lead hazards within a specified period are served on property owners. The ordered abatement work is monitored and ultimately certified as complete. Noncompliant owners can be fined substantially. In some jurisdictions, the health or housing departments are authorized to preemptively perform abatements and charge the cost as an assessment on property taxes.

STRATEGIC PREVENTION

Compelling clinical and epidemiological research published during the 1980s and 1990s established the need for a strategic, long-term campaign to eliminate childhood lead poisoning. In 1991, the CDC proposed a "Strategic Plan for the Elimination of Childhood Lead Poisoning" (U.S. Department of Health and Human Services, 1991). The CDC plan has since been augmented by broad-scope plans of other governmental agencies (U.S. Department of Housing and Urban Development, 1990; U.S. EPA, 1991). Private, nonprofit advocacy groups have offered more targeted plans (Alliance to End Childhood Lead Poisoning, 1993b; National Center for Lead Safe Housing, 1993). Common threads that run through all of them are the need for long-term planning, new funding sources, evaluation of outcomes and leadership.

Creating effective and cost-efficient models for the remediation of lead-hazardous housing ranks as one of the most pressing tasks of the mid-1990s. Many cities, with funds supplied by the Department of Housing and Urban Development, are now developing, implementing, and evaluating locally appropriate remediation models. The results of these environmental experiments were to be available in 1996. Health-based clearance standards for lead in household dust are being developed by the EPA.

However, given effective and cost-efficient remediation, there are an estimated 14 million homes in the United States that would benefit from it. Much of the work will be privately financed by the property owners, but it is likely that new sources of public funding will be required to subsidize this multi-billion–dollar endeavor. Excise taxes on lead-containing products have been proposed, and a class-action suit against paint manufacturers has been brought. It has also been proposed that, in order to stretch funding and combat poverty at the same time, community action and Job Corps programs should train and employ people to rebuild their own neighborhoods (Needleman, 1990).

Perhaps the most innovative and far-reaching of the proposals for generating the needed funds calls for fundamental reorganization of the income tax structure of the United States (Dolbeare, 1994). Dolbeare of the National Low Income Housing Coalition argues that income tax deductions granted for high-end home mortgages are an irrational subsidy of approximately $15 billion per year to that portion of the population that needs it least. Such regressive tax systems create an artificial market that rewards the construction of underused mansions for the rich at the expense of desperately needed basic housing for the poor and middle classes.

Strategic prevention connects the community-oriented work of local lead poisoning prevention programs to structural changes on the national level and directs them both toward a common goal. Progress toward the elimination of childhood lead poisoning in the United States will necessarily be incremental. Elimination is achievable, however, and ought to be accomplished during the first few years of the 21st century.

REFERENCES

Alliance to End Childhood Lead Poisoning. (1993a). *A framework for action to make private housing lead safe.* Washington, DC: Author.

Alliance to End Childhood Lead Poisoning. (1993b). *Understanding Title X: A practical guide to the Residential Lead-Based Paint Hazard Reduction Act of 1992.* Washington, DC: Author.

Amitai, Y., Brown, M.J., Graef, J.W., & Cosgrove, E. (1991). Residential deleading: Effects on the blood lead levels of lead-poisoned children. *Pediatrics, 88*(5), 893–897.

Annest, J.L., Pirkle, J.L., Makuc, D., Neese, J.W., Bayse, D.D., & Kovar, M.G. (1983). Chronological trend in blood lead levels between 1976 and 1980. *New England Journal of Medicine, 308*, 1373–1377.

Baghurst, P.A., McMichael, A.J., Wigg, N.R., Vimpani, G.V., Robertson, E.F., Roberts, R.J., & Tong, S.L. (1992). Environmental exposure to lead and children's intelligence at the age of seven years. The Port Pirie cohort study. *New England Journal of Medicine, 327,* 1279–1284.

Bellinger, D., Leviton, A., Waternaux, C., Needleman, H., & Rabinowitz, M. (1987). Longitudinal analyses of prenatal and postnatal lead exposure and early cognitive development. *New England Journal of Medicine, 316,* 1037–1043.

Billick, I.H., Curran, A.S., & Shier, D.R. (1980). Relation of pediatric blood lead levels to lead in gasoline. *Environmental Health Perspectives, 34,* 213–217.

Binns, H.J., LeBailly, S.A., Poncher, J., Kinsella, T.R., & Saunders, S.E. (1994). Is there lead in the suburbs? Risk assessment in Chicago suburban pediatric practices. *Pediatrics, 93,* 164–171.

Brody, D.J., Pirkle, J.L., Kramer, R.A., Flegal, K.M., Matte, T.D., Gunter, E.W., & Paschal, D.C. (1994). Blood lead levels in the US population. Phase one of the Third National Health and Nutrition Examination Survey (NHANES III, 1988 to 1991). *Journal of the American Medical Association, 272,* 277–283.

Brown, M.J., DeGiacomo, J.M., Gallagher, G., Graef, J., Leff, J., Mathieu, O., Nguyen, H., Petre, R., Prenney, B., & Sagov, S. (1990). Lead poisoning in children of different ages. *New England Journal of Medicine, 323,* 135–136.

Centers for Disease Control (CDC). (1988). Childhood lead poisoning—United States: Report to the Congress by the Agency for Toxic Substances and Disease Registry. *Morbidity and Mortality Weekly Report, 37,* 481–485.

Centers for Disease Control and Prevention (CDC). (1991). *Preventing lead poisoning in young children.* Atlanta, GA: Author.

Davis, J.M., & Svendsgaard, D.J. (1987). Lead and child development. *Nature, 329,* 297–300.

Dietrich, K.N., Krafft, K.M., Bornschein, R.L., Hammond, P.B., Berger, O., Succop, P.A., & Bier, M. (1987). Low-level fetal lead exposure: Effect on neurobehavioral development in early infancy. *Pediatrics, 80,* 721–730.

Dolbeare, C.N. (1994). *Working paper on federal housing trust fund proposal.* Washington, DC: National Low Income Housing Coalition.

Farfel, M.R., & Chisolm, J.J. (1990). Health and environmental outcomes of traditional and modified practices for abatement of residential lead-based paint. *American Journal of Public Health, 80,* 1240–1245.

Faust, D., & Brown, J. (1987). Moderately elevated blood lead levels: Effects on neuropsychologic functioning in children. *Pediatrics, 80,* 623–629.

Hayes, E.B., McElvaine, M.D., Orbach, H.G., Fernandez, A.M., Lyne, S., & Matte, T.D. (1994). Long-term trends in blood lead levels among children in Chicago: Relationship to air lead levels. *Pediatrics, 93,* 195–200.

Karch and Associates, Inc. (1988). Review of the biological basis of the proposed drinking water standards for lead—A summary. *Water Research Quarterly, 1,* 11–13.

Kimbrough, R.D., LeVois, M., & Webb, D.R. (1994). Management of children with slightly elevated blood lead levels. *Pediatrics, 93,* 188–191.

Landrigan, P.J. (1982). Occupational and community exposures to toxic metals: Lead, cadmium, mercury, and arsenic. *Western Journal of Medicine, 137,* 531–539.

Landrigan, P.J., & Baker, E.L. (1981). Exposure of children to heavy metals from smelters: Epidemiology and toxic consequences. *Environmental Research, 25,* 204–224.

Landrigan, P.J., Gehlbach, S.H., Rosenblum, B.F., Shoults, J.M., Candelaria, R.M., Barthel, W.F., Liddle, T.A., Smrek, A.L., Staehling, N.W., & Sanders,

J.F. (1975). Epidemic lead absorption near an ore smelter. *New England Journal of Medicine, 292,* 123–129.

Mahaffey, K.R. (1981). Nutritional factors in lead poisoning. *Nutrition Reviews, 39,* 353–362.

Mahaffey, K.R. (1983). Sources of lead in the urban environment [editorial]. *American Journal of Public Health, 73,* 1357–1358.

Mahaffey, K.R., Annest, J.L., Roberts, J., & Murphy, R.S. (1982). National estimates of blood lead levels: United States, 1976–1980: Association with selected demographic and socioeconomic factors. *New England Journal of Medicine, 307,* 573–579.

Marino, P.E., Landrigan, P.J., Graef, J., Nussbaum, A., Bayan, G., Boch, K., & Boch, S. (1990). A case report of lead paint poisoning during renovation of a Victorian farmhouse. *American Journal of Public Health, 80,* 1183–1185.

Markowitz, S.B., Nunez, C.M., Klitzman, S., Munshi, A.A., Kim, W.S., Eisinger, J., & Landrigan, P.J. (1994). Lead poisoning due to hai ge fen: The porphyrin content of individual erythrocytes. *Journal of the American Medical Association, 271,* 932–934.

McMichael, A.J., Baghurst, P.A., Wigg, N.R., Vimpani, G.V., Robertson, E.F., & Roberts, R.J. (1988). Port Pirie cohort study: Environmental exposure to lead and children's abilities at the age of four years. *New England Journal of Medicine, 319,* 468–475.

Mushak, P., & Crocetti, A.F. (1990). Methods for reducing lead exposure in young children and other risk groups: An integrated summary of a report to the U.S. Congress on childhood lead poisoning. *Environmental Health Perspectives, 89,* 125–135.

National Center for Lead Safe Housing. (1993). *Lead-based paint hazards and the comprehensive housing affordability strategy (CHAS).* Columbia, MD: Author.

Needleman, H.L. (1990). The future challenge of lead toxicity. *Environmental Health Perspectives, 89,* 85–89.

Needleman, H.L., & Gastonis, C.A. (1990). Low-level lead exposure and the IQ of children. A meta-analysis of modern studies. *Journal of the American Medical Association, 263,* 673–678.

Needleman, H.L., Gunnoe, C., Leviton, A., Reed, R., Peresie, H., Maher, C., & Barrett, P. (1979). Deficits in psychologic and classroom performance of children with elevated dentine lead levels. *New England Journal of Medicine, 300,* 689–695.

Needleman, H.L., Schell, A., Bellinger, D., Leviton, A., & Allred, E.N. (1990). The long-term effects of exposure to low doses of lead in childhood. An 11-year follow-up report. *New England Journal of Medicine, 322,* 83–88.

Nordin, J.D., Rolnick, S.J., & Griffin, J.M. (1994). Prevalence of excess lead absorption and associated risk factors in children enrolled in a midwestern health maintenance organization. *Pediatrics, 93,* 172–177.

Residential Lead-Based Paint Hazard Reduction Act of 1992, PL 102-550. (October 28, 1992). Title 42, U.S.C. §§ 1437a et seq.: *U.S. Statutes at Large, 106,* 3672–4097.

Schaffer, S.J., Szilagyi, P.G., & Weitzman, M. (1994). Lead poisoning risk determination in an urban population through the use of a standardized questionnaire. *Pediatrics, 93,* 159–163.

Schlenker, T.L. (1989). The effects of lead in Milwaukee's water. *Wisconsin Medical Journal, 88*(10), 13–15.

Schlenker, T.L. (1992a). Lead poisoning in children. The ramifications and the road to prevention. *Postgraduate Medicine, 92,* 69–74.

Schlenker, T.L. (1992b). A rationale for universal screening for childhood lead poisoning. *Wisconsin Medical Journal, 91,* 133–135.

Schlenker, T.L., Fritz, C.J., Mark, D., Layde, M., Linke, G., Murphy, A., & Matte, T. (1994). Screening for pediatric lead poisoning: Comparability of simultaneously drawn capillary and venous blood samples. *Journal of the American Medical Association, 271,* 1346–1348.

Schlenker, T.L., Fritz, C.J., Murphy, A., & Shepeard, S. (1994). Feasibility and effectiveness of screening for childhood lead poisoning in private medical practice. *Archives of Pediatric and Adolescent Medicine, 148,* 761–764.

Schwartz, J., & Pitcher, H. (1989). The relationship between gasoline lead and blood lead in the United States. *Official Statistics, 5,* 421–431.

Shannon, M.W., & Graef, J.W. (1992). Lead intoxication in infancy. *Pediatrics, 89,* 87–90.

Shukla, R., Dietrich, K.N., Bornschein, R.L., Berger, O., & Hammond, P.B. (1991). Lead exposure and growth in the early preschool child: A follow-up report from the Cincinnati lead study. *Pediatrics, 88,* 886–892.

Smith, D.C., Beller, M., & Middaugh, J.P. (1992). Lead ingestion associated with ceramic glaze. *Morbidity and Mortality Weekly Report, 41,* 781–783.

Staes, C., Matte, T., Copley, C.G., Flanders, D., & Binder, S. (1994). Retrospective study of the impact of lead-based paint hazard remediation on children's blood lead levels in St. Louis, Missouri. *American Journal of Epidemiology, 139,* 1016–1026.

Tejeda, D.M., Wyatt, D.D., Rostek, B.R., & Solomon, W.B. (1994). Do questions about lead exposure predict elevated lead levels? *Pediatrics, 93,* 192–194.

Trotter, R.T. (1990). The cultural parameters of lead poisoning: A medical anthropologist's view of intervention in environmental lead exposure. *Environmental Health Perspectives, 89,* 79–84.

U.S. Department of Health and Human Services. (1991). *Strategic plan for the elimination of childhood lead poisoning.* Atlanta, GA: CDC.

U.S. Department of Housing and Urban Development. (1990). *Comprehensive and workable plan for the abatement of lead-based paint in privately owned housing: Report to Congress.* Washington, DC: Office of Policy Development and Research.

U.S. Environmental Protection Agency (EPA). (1991). *Strategy for reducing lead exposures: Report to Congress.* Washington, DC: Author.

U.S. Food and Drug Administration (FDA), Department of Health and Human Services. (1993). Emergency action levels: Lead in food packed in lead-soldered cans. *Federal Register, 58,* 17233–17236.

Weitzman, M., Aschengrau, A., Bellinger, D., Jones, R., Hamlin, J.S., & Beiser, A. (1993). Lead-contaminated soil abatement and urban children's blood lead levels. *Journal of the American Medical Association, 269,* 1647–1654.

12

ECONOMIC ISSUES
OF CHILDHOOD
LEAD POISONING

Deborah E. Glotzer

Any discussion about the economic aspects of childhood lead poisoning should begin with mention of its epidemiology. The dramatic decrease in blood lead levels since the mid-1980s is considered to be a major public health achievement primarily due to governmental action that reduced lead exposure from multiple sources, such as gasoline and canned foods (Pirkle et al., 1994). However, despite this laudable improvement, minority, urban, and low-income children continue to have mean blood lead levels and a risk of blood lead elevation considerably higher than that of nonminority and more affluent children (Brody et al., 1994). Thus, those children already disadvantaged in terms of socioeconomic status are further disadvantaged through increased lead exposure, in large part as a result of poor housing conditions. Whether the response to household lead exposure is adequate is open to debate; some have argued that exposure would not continue if its victims were predominantly affluent and nonminority.

The economic aspects of medical and public health issues have received increased examination and focus in recent years as monetary constraints have become more acute and as health care and insurance reform continue to reshape clinical practice. Childhood lead poisoning has also become an area of increasing controversy and attention, particularly with regard to the lowering of the minimum acceptable blood lead level and the resulting recommendations for increased screening, surveillance, and management. Much of the debate about childhood lead poisoning has revolved around the costs, benefits, and effectiveness of these new recommendations, particularly in comparison with other pediatric problems. Some have argued that the increased attention and financial resources currently devoted to childhood lead poisoning would be more effectively used for other childhood problems such as premature births, child abuse, and violence in our society (Sayre & Ernhart, 1992; Schoen, 1993). These arguments are based on the premises that the adverse effects of low-level lead poisoning are clinically insignificant and that lead surveillance and management are costly, with marginal or unproven benefit. However, these sweeping statements have been made without formal cost analysis. Furthermore, although well intentioned, few programs aimed at reducing morbidity from these other problems have been subjected to scientific scrutiny or economic evaluation. In contrast, a number of issues related to the management of childhood lead poisoning have undergone formal economic evaluation.

Decision analysis has been the primary tool used to investigate the economics of various aspects of childhood lead poisoning. This chapter reviews the basics of decision analysis and economic evaluation and examines those studies that have explored the economics of childhood lead poisoning.

ECONOMIC EVALUATION AND DECISION ANALYSIS

Decision analysis is a systematic method of modeling alternative strategies. It can be used to determine which strategy is preferred for a given set of specified conditions and can identify the variables that are most important in decision making (Pauker & Kassirer, 1987). The decision model is based on the probabilities of various outcomes and the values assigned to those outcomes (Figure 1). Values (often referred to as utilities) may be measured in dollars or by clinical indices such as years of life saved (YLS) or quality-adjusted life expectancy (QALE), depending on the type of analysis. Baseline probabilities and values are derived from published data, best-guess estimates, expert opinions, hospital costs, or other sources. These allow for calculation of the model under base case conditions. There is always uncertainty under base case conditions, even in the most meticulously constructed models, because of inherent imprecision in published data or lack of hard data. Therefore, sensitivity analysis is then used to examine how the

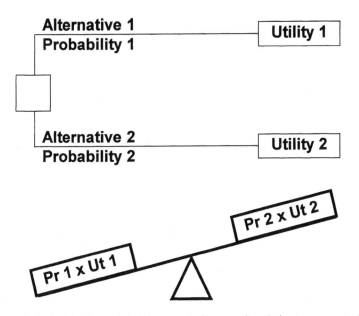

Figure 1. The basis of decision analysis. This schematic diagram outlines the basic components of decision analysis. Alternative strategies are modeled using a decision tree. The preferred strategy is identified by comparing the expected values of each decision branch. The expected value for each branch is determined by the product of the probabilities and utilities along the branch.

model output changes as probabilities and utilities are varied through their range of uncertainty.

There are three basic types of economic analysis: cost identification, cost-effectiveness and cost–benefit (Figure 2) (Eisenberg, 1989).

1. *Cost identification* analysis is used to compare the costs of alternative management options that have equivalent outcomes, such as the costs of lead screening by different strategies (Glotzer, Bauchner, Freedberg, & Palfrey, 1994).

2. *Cost-effectiveness* analysis compares the costs and outcomes of competing strategies when outcomes are measured in clinical units, such as YLS, QALE, or cases of disease. This allows comparison of the ratios of costs to outcomes among strategies, such as the cost per case of averted learning disability of lead screening by different screening tests (Berwick & Komaroff, 1982).

3. *Cost–benefit* analysis assigns an economic value to outcomes, thereby comparing costs and benefits in the same units, and explicitly examines the issue of whether the outcome is worth the costs, such as the costs and benefits of reducing the lead content of gasoline (Schwartz, Pitcher, Levin, Ostro, & Nichols, 1985).

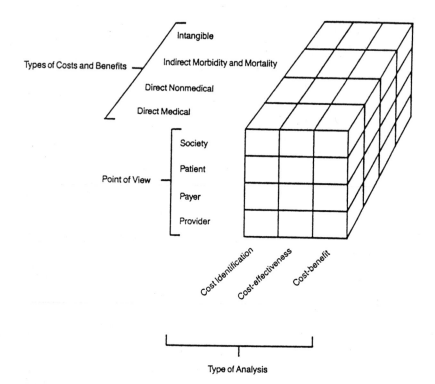

Figure 2.   Three dimensions of clinical economics. (From Eisenberg, J.M. [1989]. Clinical economics: A guide to the economic analysis of clinical practices. *Journal of the American Medical Association, 262,* 2879–2886; reprinted by permission.)

All economic analyses can be viewed from an individual or societal perspective and may include direct medical costs (e.g., hospitalization, diagnostic testing), direct nonmedical costs (e.g., educational costs, home care), indirect costs (e.g., lost income from increased morbidity and mortality), and intangible costs (e.g., pain and suffering, quality of life). In a cost–benefit analysis, intangible costs are assigned a monetary value.

ECONOMICS OF REDUCING LEAD IN GASOLINE

Public health policy and subsequently health outcomes have been shaped by the analyses described above. For example, in a 1985 report, the U.S. Environmental Protection Agency (EPA) concluded that reducing the lead content of gasoline would result in overall cost savings (Schwartz, 1994; Schwartz et al., 1985). This report examined the increased cost of reducing lead exposure through the refinement of low-lead gasoline along with the offsetting economic benefits of reduced medical and educational costs resulting from improved child health and cognitive outcome, decreased hypertension in adult males, decreased nonlead environmental pollutants from better refining techniques, and improved fuel economy. The analysis projected a net annual savings in excess of $1 billion using the most conservative estimates. An extrapolation of this study estimated an annual benefit of $3.5 billion from reduced adverse health effects alone if the mean population blood lead concentration were reduced by only 1 μg/dL (Schwartz, 1994). Following the phase-down of lead in gasoline, the mean blood lead level in the United States has decreased by 78%, from 12.8 to 2.8 μg/dL (Annest et al., 1983; Pirkle et al., 1994). The health benefit from the reduction of lead in gasoline is well accepted, and, because the magnitude of the decrease is so large, the economic benefit is considerable as well.

ECONOMICS OF LEAD PAINT ABATEMENT

Other environmental interventions to reduce lead exposure have undergone economic evaluation, but this information has not yet influenced public policy. In its 1991 strategic plan for the elimination of childhood lead poisoning, the Centers for Disease Control (CDC) focused primarily on household lead paint abatement because paint is the major pathway through which children become poisoned (Binder & Falk, 1991).

In a cost–benefit analysis, the CDC projected that lead paint abatement for an average pre-1950 home containing lead-based paint would result in a net savings of $2,098 per housing unit (in 1989 dollars) (Binder & Falk, 1991). This analysis estimated that the cost of an average abatement is $2,225 and would result in a $4,323 benefit. Abating all pre-1950 housing containing lead-based paint was estimated to save $62 billion over a 20-year period. The predicted benefits are from reduced medical and special education costs, increased future employment productivity, and reduced neonatal mortality.

The potential benefits of reducing other lead-induced adverse health effects, such as impaired growth, hearing, and hematopoiesis in children and hypertension in adults, were not included because of the difficulty in quantifying them. Similarly, the contribution of lead to juvenile delinquency, depressed property values, and an individual's emotional well-being was not considered. The omission of these factors results in an underestimation of the potential benefits of lead abatement.

The estimates of the cost and effectiveness of paint abatement used in this analysis were derived from data obtained in the late 1970s and early 1980s. Currently used abatement techniques are considerably more rigorous and expensive. Although these newer techniques are generally believed to be more effective, mid-1990s data suggest that they may be of limited effectiveness or even detrimental, depending on a child's initial blood lead level (Staes, Matte, Copley, Flanders, & Binder, 1994; Swindell, Charney, Brown, & Delaney, 1994). If in fact the effectiveness of lead paint abatement is considerably more limited and/or more costly than the estimates used in the analysis, then the model will overestimate the benefit.

ECONOMICS OF OTHER HOME-BASED ENVIRONMENTAL INTERVENTIONS TO REDUCE LEAD EXPOSURE

A 1994 study addressed the costs and benefits of other environmental interventions for children with borderline and low-level blood lead elevations (Glotzer, Weitzman, Aschengrau, & Freedberg, 1994). This cost–benefit analysis was based on data from a randomized clinical trial that investigated the effectiveness of one-time interior loose paint stabilization, interior dust abatement, and soil abatement. The analysis used the actual costs of the environmental interventions and estimated the projected costs of medical follow-up, special education, and future lifetime earnings based on pre- and postintervention blood lead levels of study participants. Because the analysis was based in large part on actual data rather than hypothetical estimates of costs and effectiveness, the empirical basis of many of the variables is strengthened. As in the CDC analysis, the financial gain of avoiding many other adverse outcomes was not considered, thus potentially underestimating the benefit of the interventions.

Under base case conditions, this analysis predicted net savings of $204 per child for loose paint stabilization plus dust abatement, and net costs of $105 and $4,761 per child for loose paint stabilization alone and for loose paint stabilization plus dust and soil abatement, respectively. Despite significant declines in blood lead levels, the soil abatement intervention appeared unlikely to be cost saving for children with low-level lead exposure, whereas net savings were projected for the paint and dust interventions under many conditions tested in the sensitivity analyses. Soil abatement would be a financially attractive strategy if the cost of abatement were substantially lower (Figure 3). Although overall cost savings is not the only criterion on which clinical and public health decisions should be made, the analy-

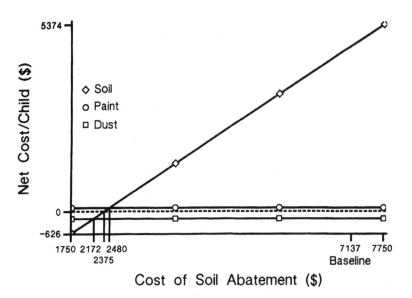

Figure 3. One-way sensitivity analysis of the cost of soil abatement versus the net cost of the soil, dust, and paint interventions. Only the cost of the soil strategy is affected, because the other interventions did not include soil abatement. Soil abatement is a financially attractive strategy only if its cost is substantially lower than the baseline value of $7,137.

sis suggested that loose paint stabilization and interior dust abatement may be a reasonable use of limited financial resources.

ECONOMICS OF SCREENING FOR CHILDHOOD LEAD POISONING

In response to the 1978 CDC guidelines for the screening, treatment, and follow-up of childhood lead poisoning, Berwick and Komaroff (1982) investigated the cost–benefit and cost effectiveness of case identification by free erythrocyte protoporphyrin (FEP) screening and blood lead measurement compared to no screening. Factors in this analysis included estimates of the prevalence of lead poisoning; sensitivity, specificity, and costs of FEP and blood lead screening; and probability and costs of lead hazard abatement, neuropsychologic sequelae, and medical management for lead-poisoned children. The monetary benefits of improved quality of life from avoided lead poisoning were not included in the model.

The model predicted that none of the strategies were cost saving under the base case assumptions. The no-screening strategy was the least expensive and least effective option, and blood lead testing was the most costly and most effective alternative (Table 1).

Table 1. Base case results for the no-screening, free erythrocyte protoporphyrin (FEP) screening, and blood lead screening strategies

Strategy	Cost of lead poisoning (per child screened)	Risk of lead-induced learning disability (no. of cases per 1,000 3-year-olds)	Risk of lead-induced mental retardation (no. of cases per 1,000 3-year-olds)
No screening	$177.80	13.37	1.41
FEP screening	$179.00	8.01	0.61
Blood lead screening	$199.10	7.05	0.60

From Berwick, D.M., & Komaroff, A.L. (1982). Cost effectiveness of lead screening. *New England Journal of Medicine, 306,* 1392–1398; reprinted by permission.

The model was particularly sensitive to changes in the base case estimates of prevalence (6.7%), effectiveness of early treatment to reduce sequelae (50%), and risk of adverse sequelae due to poisoning (2%–55%, depending on lead level). Sensitivity analysis indicated that if the prevalence of elevated lead levels (defined as ≥30 μg/dL) was 7% or higher, FEP screening was less costly and more effective than no screening (Figure 4).

Because of decreased lead exposure, the current prevalence of blood lead levels >25 μg/dL does not exceed 1.4%, even among the

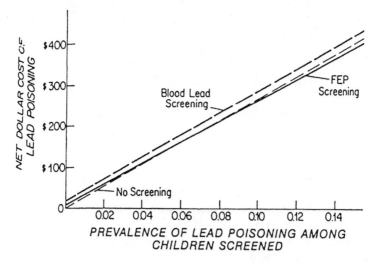

Figure 4. One-way sensitivity analysis of the prevalence of lead poisoning (defined as blood lead level ≥30 μg/dL) versus the cost of lead poisoning in 1979 dollars according to the no-screening, free erythrocyte protoporphyrin (FEP) screening, and blood lead screening strategies. The blood lead screening strategy is the most costly alternative for the range of prevalence tested. FEP screening is less costly than no screening if the prevalence of lead poisoning exceeds 7%. (From Berwick, D.M., & Komaroff, A.L. [1982]. Cost effectiveness of lead screening. *New England Journal of Medicine, 306,* 1392–1398; reprinted by permission.)

most high-risk groups (Brody et al., 1994). The effectiveness of early treatment remains an unknown, and more recent data indicate that the adverse neurocognitive sequelae may be greater than previously recognized. Therefore, it is likely that the actual cost–benefit and cost-effectiveness of the screening strategies differ from model projections. However, the conceptual model remains quite useful and could be used to evaluate the current cost–benefit and cost-effectiveness of lead screening strategies.

In 1991, DeBaun and Sox evaluated the effectiveness of FEP screening for lead poisoning (defined here as blood lead ≥25 µg/dL) with a decision model similar to that used by Berwick and Komaroff. It is well established that FEP testing is not adequately sensitive to detect many children with elevated blood lead levels, particularly those with levels <25 µg/dL (McElvaine et al., 1991). Based on the sensitivity and specificity of the FEP assay, this model predicted that no FEP threshold exists that maximizes the economic benefits of screening if the prevalence of elevated lead levels is >8%. Based on economic criteria alone, the model suggests that FEP screening may be a practical screening test if the prevalence of elevated lead levels (≥25 µg/dL) is <3%. However, the model did not consider the costs, benefits, or FEP test performance associated with identification of blood lead levels <25 µg/dL. These factors may alter this conclusion. Given the Third National Health and Nutrition Examination Survey data, which demonstrate a lower prevalence of elevated blood lead levels than those of earlier surveys (Brody et al., 1994; Pirkle et al., 1994), it seems reasonable to reconsider whether FEP screening is a rational screening strategy for areas of low prevalence.

The 1991 CDC guidelines promulgated the recommendation of universal screening with blood lead testing (CDC, 1991). The 1990 Population Survey conducted by the U.S. Bureau of the Census estimated that there are more than 18 million children in the United States under the age of 6 years; therefore, the costs of universal screening are substantial. The guidelines further advised that a level of 15 µg/dL or greater from a capillary sample should be confirmed by a venous sample because capillary samples may be falsely positive. However, obtaining specimens by venipuncture is more difficult than by capillary sampling, and initial screening by venipuncture is not as widely used (Edwards & Forsyth, 1989).

Glotzer et al. (1994) used decision analysis to investigate the cost of universal blood lead screening by three screening strategies: 1) venipuncture; 2) capillary sample with venipuncture confirmation if the blood lead level is elevated; and 3) stratification by risk, with venipuncture for high-risk children and capillary sample for low-risk children. Under base case assumptions, the cost of screening by the venipuncture, stratification, and capillary strategies was $22, $25, and $27, respectively; the capillary strategy was 23% more costly than the venipuncture strategy. Because venipuncture is the final step in all the screening strategies, and because the cost of laboratory analysis is the same for capillary and venous samples, the venipuncture strategy is the least expensive strategy, unless the cost of venipuncture phlebotomy is more than three times higher than the cost of capillary sampling (Figure 5).

This model did not consider the child and parent preferences for the sampling method and did not factor in the cost of parental time for accompanying the child. Although it may appear that initial screening by capillary sample rather than venipuncture is simpler, that may not be true if a confirmatory venipuncture sample is required.

The model was sensitive to changes in the base case estimates of costs of blood lead analysis and phlebotomy, prevalence of elevated blood lead levels, and false-positive rate for capillary specimens. Mid-1990s data indicate that the base case estimates of the prevalence of elevated levels and the false-positive rate used in the model may be too high (Brody et al., 1994; Schlenker et al., 1994). If these more recent estimates are used, the model indicates that the capillary or stratification strategies would be less expensive than the venipuncture strategy. It is likely that the optimal screening strategy will differ by commun-

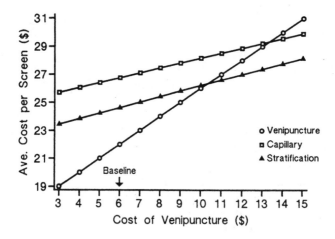

Figure 5.   Cost of lead screening as a function of cost of venipuncture. Venipuncture is the least expensive strategy unless its cost exceeds $10 per sample. The capillary strategy is more costly than the venipuncture strategy if the cost of venipuncture is less than $13 per sample. In the baseline analysis, the costs of venipuncture and capillary sampling were $6 and $3 per sample, respectively. (From Glotzer, D.E., Bauchner, H., Freedberg, K.A., & Palfrey, S. [1994]. Screening for childhood lead poisoning: A cost-minimization analysis. *American Journal of Public Health, 84,* 110–112; reprinted by permission.)

ity, based on the local prevalence of elevated blood lead levels, costs of laboratory analysis and phlebotomy, and the false-positive rate of capillary sampling under nonstudy conditions.

COST-EFFECTIVENESS OF CHELATION FOR ELEVATED BLOOD LEAD LEVELS

The decision models that evaluated the cost–benefit of lead screening included the assumption that children with elevated blood lead levels would receive chelation therapy, but the models did not assess the impact of treatment for children identified to have an elevated blood lead level, independent of the effectiveness of screening to detect elevated levels (Berwick & Komaroff, 1982; DeBaun & Sox, 1991). No consensus exists regarding the preferred treatment strategy for low-level childhood lead poisoning, and a substantial fraction of pediatricians do not recommend chelation for such children (Glotzer & Bauchner, 1992). Lead treatment strategies differ in the incidence and severity of adverse drug effects, inconvenience associated with treatment, treatment costs, and, possibly, cognitive outcomes. In a cost-effectiveness analysis, Glotzer, Freedberg, and Bauchner (1995) investigated the trade-offs of these factors with a model that was based on a 2-year-old child with newly identified moderate lead poisoning (blood lead level 25–39 µg/dL).

The model compared the clinical impact and cost-effectiveness of four treatment strategies: 1) no treatment (NO RX); 2) calcium disodium ethylenediaminetetraacetic acid (EDTA) provocation testing, followed by chelation if testing is positive (PROV); 3) penicillamine chelation with crossover to EDTA provocation testing if toxicity occurs (PCA); and 4) EDTA provocation testing with crossover to penicillamine chelation if testing is negative (EDTA) (Figure 6).

In the baseline analysis, it was assumed that, in children whose blood lead levels were successfully reduced by chelation, the risk of developing a reading disability as a result of lead exposure decreased by 70%. Under the baseline conditions tested, the PCA and EDTA strategies were substantially more effective than the NO RX and PROV strategies in terms of the number of reading disability cases prevented and in quality-adjusted life years gained. For example, the PCA and EDTA strategies prevented 22.5% of cases of reading disability and increased QALE by 1.02 years compared with no treatment.

Under most conditions tested in the sensitivity analyses, the cost per case of reading disability prevented by the PROV, EDTA, and PCA strategies compared with no treatment is far less than the estimated

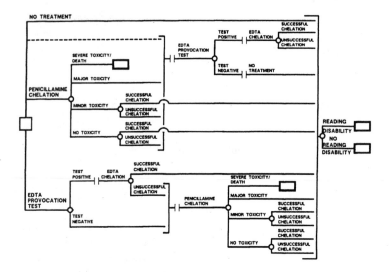

Figure 6. Decision model for treatment of childhood lead poisoning. See text for explanation of management strategies. Square nodes represent decisions; circular nodes represent chance occurrences; double lines represent label nodes; rectangular nodes represent outcomes; brackets indicate that branches ending at bracket enter subtrees depicted to right of bracket. Broken line indicates that strategy begins with ethylenediaminetetraacetic acid (EDTA) provocation test (From Glotzer, D.E., Freedberg, K.A., & Bauchner, H. [1995]. Management of childhood lead poisoning: Clinical impact and cost-effectiveness. *Medical Decision Making, 15,* 13–24; reprinted by permission.)

cost of remedial education (Table 2). This indicated that the PROV, EDTA, and PCA strategies are all cost saving compared with no treatment when educational costs are considered. Even if remedial education costs are not considered, the EDTA and PCA strategies are at least as cost-effective as many medical interventions that are generally accepted for widespread use.

The effectiveness of chelation in preventing neuropsychological morbidity, such as a reading disability, is not known. This decision model indicates that even if chelation reduced the risk of lead-induced reading disability by only 12%–20%, depending on treatment strategy, it would be cost saving (Figure 7). This model did not consider indirect costs of lead poisoning, such as decreased future lifetime earnings through reductions in wage rate and labor force participation. Therefore, the monetary benefits estimated from the model are conservative.

Because a number of the assumptions used in the model are not based on conclusive data, the results should not be viewed as a prescription for treatment. However, it appears that chelation of lead-poisoned children is likely to have both economic and clinical benefits.

Table 2. Sensitivity analysis

Variable (baseline value, value tested)	Strategies[a]	Cost ($)	Cost/case prevented ($)[b]	Incremental cost-effectiveness ratio[c] ($/case prevented)
Cost: remedial education ($0, $27,614)	EDTA	7,748	−21,763[d]	—
	PCA	8,001	−20,633	Dominated[e]
	PROV	10,540	−23,923	Dominated
	NO RX	12,636	—	Dominated
Cost: penicillamine chelation ($1,632, $800)	NO RX	463	—	—
	PROV	786	3,688	Extended dominance[f]
	PCA	1,200	3,281	3,281
	EDTA	1,232	3,421	Dominated
Cost: EDTA provocation test ($238, $600)	NO RX	463	—	—
	PROV	1,148	7,821	Extended dominance
	PCA	2,099	7,280	7,280
	EDTA	2,140	7,466	Dominated
Cost: EDTA chelation ($506, $2,500)	NO RX	463	—	—
	PROV	1,484	11,656	Extended dominance
	PCA	2,160	7,553	7,553
	EDTA	2,476	8,962	Dominated
Probability of positive EDTA provocation test (355, 105)	NO RX	463	—	—
	PROV	726	10,481	Extended dominance
	PCA	2,021	7,308	7,308
	EDTA	2,087	7,618	Dominated

From Glotzer, D.E., Freedberg, K.A., & Bauchner, H. (1995). Management of childhood lead poisoning: Clinical impact and cost-effectiveness. *Medical Decision Making, 15*, 13–24; reprinted by permission.

[a] Strategies listed in order of increasing cost: NO RX = no treatment; PROV = EDTA provocation test, with no treatment if test result is negative; EDTA = EDTA provocation test with crossover to penicillamine if test result is negative; PCA = penicillamine chelation with crossover to EDTA provocation test if toxicity occurs.

[b] Compared with no-treatment strategy.

[c] Incremental cost-effectiveness ratios indicate the additional cost per additional case of reading disability prevented using a more costly and more effective strategy.

[d] Negative numbers indicate that EDTA, PCA, and PROV strategies are cost saving when costs of remedial education are included.

[e] Dominated indicates that strategy is not cost-effective compared with the next less expensive strategy because of higher costs and equal or lower effectiveness.

[f] Extended dominance indicates that strategy is not cost-effective compared with next more expensive strategy because it has a higher incremental cost-effectiveness ratio. The more expensive strategy is associated with more effectiveness for a fixed cost.

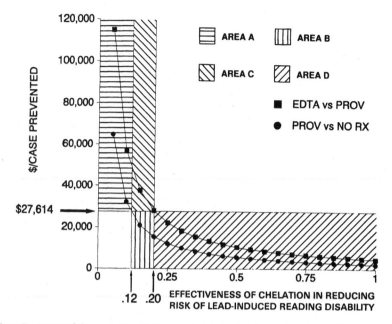

Figure 7.   Impact of changes in the effectiveness of chelation in reducing the risk of lead-induced read-ing disability on the incremental cost-effectiveness of the EDTA and provocation test strategies. The cost of medical treatment exceeds the cost of remedial education ($27,614) only if chelation reduces the risk of reading disability by less than 12% (area A). The cost of preventing lead-induced reading disability with the EDTA strategy exceeds the cost of remedial education if the effectiveness of chelation is between 12% and 20% (area B). If chelation effectiveness is between 12% and 20%, the cost of prevent-ing a case of reading disability with the provocation test strategy is less than the cost of remedial educa-tion (area C). If chelation effectiveness is 20% or greater, the EDTA strategy is cost saving compared to all other strategies if costs of remedial education are considered (area D). (From Glotzer, D.E., Freedberg, K.A., & Bauchner, H. [1995]. Management of childhood lead poisoning: Clinical impact and cost-effectiveness. *Medical Decision Making, 15,* 19; reprinted by permission.)

CONCLUSIONS

Many would argue that lead poisoning is the most serious environ-mental threat to this nation's children. The prevention and treatment of elevated lead exposure during childhood are complex medical and public health issues. The economic impact of a number of lead preven-tion and treatment strategies has been examined. Although the specific conclusions reached through these economic evaluations may change as new data are generated, the methodology remains sound and the decision models provide a useful framework to help develop a rational plan to address childhood lead exposure, especially if the resources for the screening, prevention, and treatment of childhood lead poisoning are limited.

REFERENCES

Annest, J.L., Pirkle, J.L., Makuc, D., Neese, J.W., Bayse, D.D., & Kovar, M.G. (1983). Chronological trend in blood lead levels between 1976 and 1980. *New England Journal of Medicine, 308*, 1373–1377.

Berwick, D.M., & Komaroff, A.L. (1982). Cost effectiveness of lead screening. *New England Journal of Medicine, 306*, 1392–1398.

Binder, S., & Falk, H. (1991). *Strategic plan for the elimination of childhood lead poisoning.* Washington, DC: U.S. Department of Health and Human Services.

Brody, D.J., Pirkle, J.L., Kramer, R.A., Flegal, K.M., Matte, T.D., Gunter, E.W., & Paschal, D.C. (1994). Blood lead levels in the U.S. population: Phase 1 of the Third National Health and Nutrition Examination Survey (NHANES III, 1988 to 1991). *Journal of the American Medical Association, 272*, 277–283.

Centers for Disease Control (CDC). (1991). *Preventing lead poisoning in young children.* Washington, DC: U.S. Department of Health and Human Services.

DeBaun, M.R., & Sox, H.C. (1991). Setting the optimal erythrocyte protoporphyrin screening decision threshold for lead poisoning: A decision analytic approach. *Pediatrics, 88*, 121–131.

Edwards, K.S., & Forsyth, B.W.C. (1989). Lead screening at pediatric teaching programs. *American Journal of Diseases of Children, 143*, 1455–1457.

Eisenberg, J.M. (1989). Clinical economics: A guide to the economic analysis of clinical practices. *Journal of the American Medical Association, 262*, 2879–2886.

Glotzer, D.E., & Bauchner, H. (1992). Management of childhood lead poisoning: A survey. *Pediatrics, 89*, 614–618.

Glotzer, D.E., Bauchner, H., Freedberg, K.A., & Palfrey, S. (1994). Screening for childhood lead poisoning: A cost-minimization analysis. *American Journal of Public Health, 84*, 110–112.

Glotzer, D.E., Freedberg, K.A., & Bauchner, H. (1995). Management of childhood lead poisoning: Clinical impact and cost-effectiveness. *Medical Decision Making, 15*, 13–24.

Glotzer, D.E., Weitzman, M., Aschengrau, A., & Freedberg, K.A. (1994). Economic evaluation of environmental interventions for low-level childhood lead poisoning. *Archives of Pediatrics and Adolescent Medicine, 148* (from Ambulatory Pediatric Association Program and Abstracts, 1994, Abstr. No. 107).

McElvaine, M.D., Orbach, H.G., Binder, S., Blanksma, L.A., Maes, E.F., & Krieg, R.M. (1991). Evaluation of the erythrocyte protoporphyrin test as a screen for elevated blood lead levels. *Pediatrics, 119*, 548–550.

Pauker, S.G., & Kassirer, J.P. (1987). Decision analysis. *New England Journal of Medicine, 316*, 250–258.

Pirkle, J.L., Brody, D.J., Gunter, E.W., Kramer, R.A., Paschal, D.C., Flegal, K.M., & Matte, T.D. (1994). The decline in blood lead levels in the United States: The National Health and Nutrition Examination Surveys (NHANES). *Journal of the American Medical Association, 272*, 284–291.

Sayre, J.W., & Ernhart, C.B. (1992). Control of lead exposure in childhood: Are we doing it correctly? [Editorial]. *American Journal of Diseases of Children, 146*, 1275–1277.

Schlenker, T.L., Fritz, C.J., Mark, D., Layde, M., Linke, G., Murphy, A., & Matte, T. (1994). Screening for pediatric lead poisoning: Comparability of simultaneously drawn capillary and venous blood samples. *Journal of the American Medical Association, 271,* 1346–1348.

Schoen, E.J. (1993). Childhood lead poisoning: Definitions and priorities. *Pediatrics, 91,* 504–506.

Schwartz, J. (1994). Societal benefits of reducing lead exposure. *Environmental Research, 66,* 105–124.

Schwartz, J., Pitcher, H., Levin, R., Ostro, B., & Nichols, A.L. (1985). *Costs and benefits of reducing lead in gasoline: Final regulatory impact analysis* (EPA-230-05-85-006). Washington, DC: U.S. Environmental Protection Agency, Office of Policy Analysis.

Staes, C., Matte, T., Copley, C.G., Flanders, D., & Binder, S. (1994). Retrospective study of the impact of lead-based paint hazard remediation on children's blood lead levels in St. Louis, Missouri. *American Journal of Epidemiology, 139,* 1016–1026.

Swindell, S.L., Charney, E., Brown, M.J., & Delaney, J. (1994). Home abatement and blood lead changes in children with class III lead poisoning. *Clinical Pediatrics,* 536–541.

INDEX

Page numbers followed by *"f"* or *"t"* indicate figures or tables, respectively.

cost-effectiveness analysis, 217,
218f
cost identification analysis,
217, 218f
gasoline, reducing lead in,
218–219
health care reform and, 215
home-based environmental interventions, 220, 221f
paint, abatement of, 219–220
screening, 221–224
free erythrocyte protoporphyrin, 222t, 222f, 223
universal blood lead, 223–224
capillary, 223–224, 224f
stratification, 223–224, 224f
venipuncture, 223–224,
224f
see also Epidemiology
Edetate calcium disodium
(CaNa₂EDTA), use of in
chelation, 151t, 152t,
153–154
Education, parental, 164
Elimination of Lead-Based Paint
Hazards in HUD-Associ-
ated Housing, and
paint, 189–190,
194–195
"Entrapado," 5
Environmental history, taking,
52–53, 53t
Epidemiology
asymptomatic children and
screening, 18–19
blood lead levels, see Blood lead
levels
exposure
low-level, effects observed at,
17–21
in shed deciduous teeth,
20–21
neurologic sequelae, 17–18
sources of, 17
Etiology, 37–53
environment
air, ambient, 38–40
bone mobilization, 48, 48t
congenital/perinatal exposure,
47–48
breastfeeding, 48
dust
abatement of, 175

inspection of, 166–167
"folk" sources
cosmetics, 49
therapeutic agents, 48–49,
49t
food, 40–42, 41t
canned, 41, 41t, 144
home-grown vegetables,
41–42, 41t
storage in lead-containing
vessels, 41, 41t
foreign bodies, 49–50, 49t
hobbies, 49, 49t
paint, see Paint
soil
abatement of, 44–45,
175–177
inspection of, 166–167
pica, 44–45
water
abatement of, 177–178
alkalinization of, 42
drinking fountains in
schools, 43
infant formula and, 43–44,
43t, 44t
inspection of, 167–168
maximum containment lev-
els, 42
plumbing, unsafe, 42–43
Safe Drinking Water Act, 42
risk factors
age, 50–51
developmental delay, 51–52
pica and, 51
nutrition
calcium deficiency and, 51
iron deficiency and, 51
pica, 51
Excretion, of lead
fecal, 151, 151t
urinary, 151, 151t
Exposure patterns, 52
paint, effect of on, see Paint

Franklin, Benjamin, 5, 10

Galena, see Lead acetate
"Gasoline huffing," 75
Gasoline, leaded, 38–40, 39f–40f
Glazing compounds, 6

Water, drinking, abatement of lead
    in—*continued*
  procedures for, 177–178
  timing of, 177
alkalinization of, 42
drinking fountains in schools, 43
infant formula and, 43–44, 43*t*–44*t*

inspection of for lead in,
    167–168
maximum containment levels, 42
plumbing, unsafe, 42–43
Safe Drinking Water Act, 42
"West India dry gripes," 5